SOMATIC EXERCISES
for Nervous System Regulation

Maya Vale

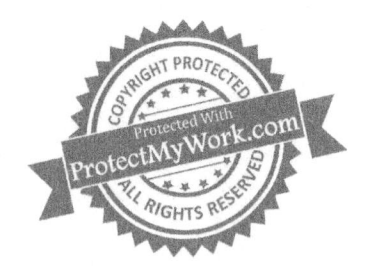

Copyright © 2025 by Maya Vale - All rights reserved.

This book and the contents herein are protected by international copyright laws. The book or any portion thereof may not be reproduced or used in any manner whatsoever without the express written permission of the publisher or author, except for the use of brief quotations in a book review or scholarly journal.

Unauthorized usage, duplication, or redistribution of this book or its content, including, but not limited to, digital copies, audio, video, electronic, photocopying, recording, or through any information storage and retrieval system, is strictly prohibited. Any infringement of this copyright notice will be liable for prosecution to the fullest extent of the law.

DISCLAIMER

The information provided within this book is for general informational purposes only. While the author has made every attempt to provide accurate, up-to-date, and complete information, the author makes no representations or warranties, express or implied, as to the accuracy, reliability, or completeness of the information contained within.

The author is not responsible for any errors or omissions, or for any actions or decisions taken based on the information provided in this book. The reader is advised to perform their own independent research and consult with a professional advisor before making any decisions based on the information provided in this book.

This book is sold with the understanding that the author is not engaged in rendering legal, financial, medical, or other professional services. If expert assistance is required, please seek the services of a competent professional.

The author assumes no responsibility for any potential damages the reader may incur in relation to the misuse of the information contained within this book. **IMAGE USAGE DISCLAIMER**

The author has made every attempt to use images that require no attribution and were sourced from credible websites. If any images are found to be used inappropriately or without the necessary permissions, please contact the author to rectify the situation promptly. The author takes no credit for any of the images used unless otherwise noted.

TABLE OF CONTENTS

Video Course and Tracking Journal Included VII

Introduction IX

Chapter 1: What is Somatic Exercise 1
    The Science Behind Somatic Exercises 2
        The Principles of Somatic Exercises 2
            Mindfulness 2
            Body Awareness 3
            Gentle Movement 3
            Resourcing 4
            Tracking 4
            Containment 5

Chapter 2: Getting Started With Somatic Exercises 7
    Preparing Your Space and Mind 7
        Tips for Selecting and Organizing Your Practice Space 8
        Essential Equipment and Attire 9
        Essential Equipment and Attire for Somatic Practice 9
        Recommendations for Selecting Yoga Mats and Props 11
    Props 11
        Tips for Choosing Comfortable Clothing for Somatic Practice 13
            Prioritize Comfort 13
            Opt for Breathable Fabrics 13
    Setting Realistic Goals 14

Chapter 3: The Forms of Somatic Exercises 17
    The History of Somatic Exercise 17
        How Somatics Work on the Nervous System 18
        The Role of the Nervous System in Stress, Anxiety, and Tension 20
            The Stress Response 20
            Anxiety: When the Alarm Gets Stuck 21
            Chronic Tension 22
        The Potential for Relief 23

Pioneers of Somatic Exercise: Hanna, Feldenkrais, and Alexander 24
    Moshe Feldenkrais: The Physicist of Movement 26
    F.M. Alexander: The Posture Pioneer 26
    The Common Thread 26

Chapter 4: Managing Anxiety with Somatic Exercise 29

Understanding Anxiety and Its Triggers 29
    Somatic Movement for Anxiety Relief 31
Breathing Techniques for Anxiety Management 47
    Box Breathing (Square Breathing) 47
    4-7-8 Breathing 47
    Alternate Nostril Breathing (Nadi Shodhana) 48
    Deep Belly Breathing (Diaphragmatic Breathing) 48

Chapter 5: Stress Relief Through Somatic Exercise 51

External and Internal Stressors 51
    External Stressors 51
    Internal Stressors 52
    Techniques for Identifying Your Personal Stressors 53
        The Body Scan Method 53
        The Stress Journal 53
        The "What If" Game 53
        The Energy Audit 54
        The Mindful Pause 54
        The Trusted Friend Perspective 54
        The Values Checklist 55
    Somatic Exercises for Relaxation 55

Chapter 6: Tension Release and Trauma Management Exercises 77

Why Tension Occurs 77
Symptoms of Tension 78
    Physical Symptoms: 78
    Emotional Symptoms: 78
    Cognitive Symptoms: 79
    Behavioral Symptoms: 79
    Somatic Movement for Tension Release 80
Foam Rolling for Tension 100

Chapter 7: 5-Minute Somatic Exercises 103

5-Minute Somatic Exercise Plans for Anxiety 103
    Grounding Breath and Body Scan 103
    Tension Release Sequence 104

Mindful Movement 105
Calming Hand and Foot Focus 105
5-Minute Somatic Exercise Plans for Stress 105
Breath and Spine Release 105
Grounding and Releasing 106
Tension Melting Sequence 106
Mindful Stretching 107
Energy Shift 107
5-Minute Somatic Exercise Plans for Trauma 107
Grounding and Present-Moment Awareness Sequence 107
Breath and Movement Connection Sequence 108
Safe Space Visualization and Anchoring 109
Important Notes: 109

Epilogue 111
Exercise List 112
Additional Reading 114

Video Course and Tracking Journal Included

Before you start! I've got something special for you: A bonus package that complements and expands on the exercises you will learn in this book. Designed to support your ongoing practice, this bonus package helps you integrate somatic awareness into your daily life.

Use your smartphone's camera to scan the QR code below, and you will be directed to a secure download page where you will receive a Google Drive link to the workbook and a Vimeo link for a more visual interpretation of the exercises.

Here is what is included in your bonus package:

- A video course for the somatic exercises covered in the book.
- A tracking journal integrating what you've learned into your daily routine and much more!

This content has been designed to support you as you continue to explore, grow, and deepen your connection with your body's wisdom.

Happy exploring, and may your somatic journey be rich and rewarding!

https://aredpen.com/sen

INTRODUCTION

Yes, you've heard it before: "Listen to your body." But, seriously—what does that even mean?

Take a second. Close your eyes if it helps. What comes up when you think about tuning into your body? Maybe it's hunger pangs or neck ache after a marathon of emails. Maybe you feel your heart go into overdrive before a big meeting. These are all valid, of course, but there's a lot more going on than just the obvious stuff.

You're probably juggling a mountain of things—work, family, and pretending you have a social life—it can feel like a circus with no ring master. The idea of "listening to your body" can feel overwhelming: one more item on a to-do list that already has a mind of its own. I get it. Believe me, I've been there. But here's your reality check: You can't keep speeding through life like it's some sort of race and expect your body to just hit the brakes when it needs to. Your body doesn't have that kind of control.

How many times do you bounce from one task to the next, only to collapse at the end of the day, wondering why you can't unwind? Stress isn't like flipping a light switch. Your body needs more than just a quick "relax already" to turn it off. It needs time. It needs care. It needs a few tricks up its sleeve to find balance.

That's where somatic therapy swoops in. It's not the same as your typical therapy session—it's more like giving your body a chance to remind you of all the wisdom it's been quietly holding on to. Somatic therapy isn't here to pile on more work. It's about equipping you with simple, science-backed tools that can slip right into your hectic life. These tools let you tap into your body's ability to reset itself—like a human version of hitting 'refresh' on your browser.

The best part? These exercises are designed for your life. No need to clear your calendar for a full-on spa day. Most of these practices take just a couple of minutes—whether you're sitting at your desk, standing in line at the store, or lying in bed trying to figure out why sleep is being so elusive.

You'll learn how your mind and body aren't just roommates—they actually need to work together. You'll understand why that connection is crucial for your mental health and how you can use it to your advantage. Plus, you'll learn simple, no-fuss exercises that help reduce stress, tame anxiety, and make you feel like you've got this whole "well-being" thing under control.

Chapter 1: What is Somatic Exercise

The human body is not an instrument to be used but a realm of one's being to be experienced, explored, enriched, and, thereby, educated—
Thomas Hannah

Buddhists view the body as more than just a shell. It's a tool for liberation, a vessel guiding us toward enlightenment and inner peace. It's not separate from us or something to dominate—it's a wise companion. Modern somatic practices echo this ancient wisdom, reminding us that our bodies store knowledge. If we pay attention, every ache, breath, and muscle twitch has a lesson or a story to tell.

The worst part is that most of us no longer possess that wisdom. In the hustle and bustle of everyday life, we ignore our bodies, push stress to the side, and push through exhaustion. Deadlines? Obligations? They're the priority. We've mastered ignoring our bodies' cues, often to our own detriment. That's where somatic exercises come in—a reset, a way to reconnect with the body we've neglected. It's about remembering how to hear what it's been trying to tell us all along.

Somatic comes from the Greek word 'soma,' meaning 'living body.' When we talk about somatic exercises, we're referring to approaches that engage the entire self—body, mind, and spirit. The mind and body aren't just roommates. They're intertwined, constantly influencing each other. Somatic exercises are the practices that use the body as a gateway to overall well-being. They're about developing body awareness, releasing tension, and learning to regulate the nervous system through mindful movement and breathing. It can be as simple as focusing on your breath or stretching gently. It can entail observing the physical signs that stress leaves behind or investigating how emotions show themselves in your body. The objective is to live in the present, listen to your body, and become in sync with it.

Somatic activities aren't just for exercising. It's working in. It's about tuning in to your internal landscape—recognizing stress signals early, being mindful of your body's needs, and living with greater embodiment in your day-to-day life.

Now, let's bring back that Buddhist idea: your body isn't just a vehicle—it's a powerful tool for transformation. When you listen to it and work with it, you're restoring the vital resources that sustain you. Those resources will fuel your peace, your resilience, and your well-being in every part of your life.

The Science Behind Somatic Exercises

To change how we feel, we need to get familiar with how we feel—especially inside. Bessel van der Kolk, in his book The Body Keeps the Score, explains that trauma and stress aren't just mental; they're physical. They live in the body. When we engage with what's happening in our body—our sensations, movements, rhythms—we're rewiring the nervous system. This creates lasting shifts in our emotional and mental state.

The power behind somatic exercises lies in neuroplasticity—the brain's ability to rewire itself. Every time we practice mindfulness and move with intention, we're forming new neural connections. These new pathways replace old patterns of stress and reactivity with calmer, more regulated responses. Studies show that mindfulness and body-based practices can even change the structure of the brain, especially areas that deal with emotional regulation, self-awareness, and stress response.

Somatic exercises don't just stop at the brain. They also directly engage the autonomic nervous system, which controls our fight-flight-freeze responses. The nervous system is shifted from a state of high alert (sympathetic activation) to one of rest and digestion (parasympathetic activation) by directing the body through particular motions and breathing patterns. This transition is essential for stress and anxiety management because it allows our bodies to rest, repair, and think clearly. It's what enables us to deal with difficulties without becoming angry or losing our composure.

The Principles of Somatic Exercises

A nervous system at ease? That's the bedrock of well-being. It's the place where your body feels safe, your mind is clear, and you engage with life from a space of completeness. Somatic exercises are the way back to a regulated nervous system and overall wellness. These exercises are rooted in core principles that work together to boost both physical and mental health. Let's break these down, no fluff:

Mindfulness

Mindfulness is the skill of being present. It's about observing your thoughts, emotions, and body sensations as they come up—no judgment, just pure awareness. It's the backbone of all somatic practices because it lets you:

- Tune in to your body's subtle signals
- Notice how your thoughts and emotions respond to situations
- Approach your experiences without reacting
- Deepen the connection between your mind and body

In action, this looks like:

- Sitting for a moment and observing your breath, no need to alter it
- Scanning your body for sensations without labeling them as good or bad
- Watching your thoughts and emotions come and go without getting tangled in them

Body Awareness

Body awareness means being attuned to your body. It's about noticing the shifts in your muscles, temperature, movements, and tension. When you develop body awareness, you catch stress before it takes hold and know how to act.

This includes:

- Recognizing where tension or relaxation shows up
- Noticing how your posture affects your mood
- Paying attention to your breathing patterns
- Sensing how emotions physically show up in your body

For example, you might realize that when you're anxious, your shoulders tense up. Or, when you're happy, there's a warm sensation in your chest. This awareness acts like an early warning system for stress, guiding you toward better self-regulation.

Gentle Movement

Somatic exercises often involve slow, deliberate movement. These aren't about pushing your body to extremes. It's about exploring what your body can do right now. Gentle movement is key to releasing tension, improving flexibility, and expanding your range of motion. Here's how you approach it:

- Move slowly and with purpose
- Stay within your comfort zone
- Focus on the quality of the movement, not how far you can push it
- Use your breath to guide the movement

For instance, try slowly rolling your shoulders, paying attention to the sensations that arise. Or take a mindful walk, focusing on the feeling of your feet making contact with the ground.

Resourcing

Your capacity to control yourself and use healthy coping strategies is known as resourcefulness. When you feel like your boat is ready to capsize due to a storm in life, it serves as your anchor. Consider it your personal health toolkit, ready and waiting for you to regain equilibrium.

Resources come in two types: external and internal.

1. **External:** External resources are people, places, pets, or activities that bring comfort and a sense of safety. It could be a friend's calming voice, a place that feels like home, the soothing presence of a pet curled up beside you, or a hobby that pulls you back to joy.

2. **Internal:** The soothing feelings or emotional states that you can access within yourself are known as internal resources. It could be the sensation of your feet firmly planted on the earth, the warmth emanating from your chest, or a recollection of a moment when you felt invincible and in control of the universe.

In somatic practice, you'll get to know these resources well. You'll learn how to identify them and make them easy to access, so when things get rocky, you've got the stability to weather the storm.

Tracking

Tracking in somatic exercises is about tuning into your body's sensations without getting caught up in a frenzy of panic, fear, or judgment. It's not about fixing anything. It's about seeing what's going on with your body, acknowledging it, and letting it be without reacting.

Effective tracking is all about cultivating a curious, non-judgmental observation of your body's rhythms. You're not trying to change anything; you're simply noticing what's happening in your body, moment by moment. This could look like:

- Scanning over your body and identifying any tense or relaxed spots
- Taking note of the depth, shallowness, speed, and steadiness of your breathing
- Paying attention to minor changes, such as tingling or temperature changes
- Observing the bodily manifestations of your emotions

Remembering that these feelings are normal is crucial when tracking. You're not in danger, even if the sensations feel intense. The goal is to approach these feelings without fear, which ultimately helps calm your nervous system over time.

Containment

One way to conceptualize containment is by building a robust wall around your emotional experiences that is both powerful enough to keep them from blowing out of control and flexible enough to let you feel them fully. It is the capacity to maintain emotional stability, feel what you are feeling, and avoid becoming enmeshed in excessive emotional spirals or reactionary behaviors.

To practice containment, you'll want to:

- Acknowledge and recognize your emotions and sensations without resistance
- Establish a boundary around the experience so it doesn't flood you
- Regulate the intensity of these sensations by focusing on what's happening right now
- Use grounding techniques, like focusing on your feet or your breath, to stay steady

Containment doesn't mean shutting down your emotions. It's about holding space for them—giving them room to exist without being overwhelmed by them. When you can do this, you process your emotions with intention, responding to life's challenges with calm and clarity.

Chapter 2: Getting Started With Somatic Exercises

Your body is the ground metaphor of your life, the expression of your existence—Gabrielle Roth

They say that the more you move, the more you understand your body. But hold on—this isn't just about moving your limbs like a wind-up toy on autopilot. No, no. This is about tuning into the subtle hum of your body's language. It's a language that's been whispering to you, patiently, all along—like a secret only you can hear when you really pay attention.

Remember that knot of tension in your shoulders after a long day? Or that butterfly dance in your stomach when excitement sneaks up on you? These sensations? They're not random. They're your body's way of sending you a message, a memo written in muscle tension, heartbeat, and breath. Somatic exercises teach us how to decipher these messages—not just hear them, but really understand what they mean—and how to respond in ways that bring your body back to balance.

We're about to start a conversation with your body. But don't expect it to be a one-sided lecture. Instead, we'll ease into gentle movements and awareness practices that anyone—yes, anyone—can do, no matter their fitness level or physical ability. The goal isn't about achieving some zen-perfect pose or pushing your body beyond its limits. Nope. The goal is far deeper: It's about learning to connect with yourself on a whole new level, recognizing your body's needs, and tapping into the endless well of wisdom it's holding.

So, as we embark on this journey, bring curiosity and patience. Your body isn't just a vessel—it's a living, breathing storybook. And it's ready to tell you its story, one sensation at a time. It's shaped by everything you've been through: your triumphs, your struggles, your moments of brilliance. Now? It's time to listen.

Preparing Your Space and Mind

The human mind doesn't just need food for thought—it needs beauty. That's why we crave aesthetically pleasing environments. It's not just about the visual appeal. It's about how beauty connects to our well-being. The right space can act like a signal to your brain that it's time to slow down, to focus, to be. And when you create that kind of space, you're giving yourself permission to sink into your somatic practice and find balance.

Your practice space doesn't need to be an Instagram-worthy yoga studio. Nope. It just needs to be a space that feels right for you—a small corner, a quiet nook, or a peaceful patch near a window. It's your sacred space, where your body knows it can come home to itself. It's about setting up a place where your mind and body can unwind from the chaos of daily life and ease into a moment of mindful awareness.

When your space supports your practice, you'll transition from the everyday rush into that sweet zone of calm with far less effort. You'll be ready to step fully into your practice, to listen closely, and to let your body show you what it's been waiting to say.

Tips for Selecting and Organizing Your Practice Space

When you're selecting your sacred space for somatic exercises, think of it as curating your own private sanctuary. Here's how to do it correctly:

- **Choose a quiet location**: Find a spot that's free from distractions. It could be a spare room, a comfortable nook in your bedroom, or, if you're feeling daring, an outdoor area where the pace of life slows down.

- **Ensure adequate space**: You don't need a ballroom, but you should have enough room to stretch out, roll around, and move freely. Think about the size of a yoga mat—perfect for your body's needs.

- **Optimize comfort**: The floor should be kind to your body. No hard, unforgiving surfaces here. Use a yoga mat, soft blanket, or carpet for a cushion that invites relaxation.

- **Control the temperature**: Comfort is king. A space that's too hot or too cold will distract you. Find a sweet spot where your body can truly relax.

- **Manage lighting**: Natural light is the ultimate. But if that's not on your side, choose soft, warm lighting to create a cozy vibe. Avoid harsh overheads—your practice isn't a spotlight audition.

- **Minimize visual clutter**: A messy space can mess with your head. Keep it free from distractions.

- **Add soothing components**: Bring in the natural world. A simple water fountain, plants, or calming artwork can all help to create a peaceful and tranquil atmosphere.

- **Have props ready**: Pillows, blankets, bolsters—keep them close by so you're not scrambling mid-practice.

CHAPTER 2: GETTING STARTED WITH SOMATIC EXERCISES

- **Create a scent-scape**: The icing on the cake for a mindful practice is aromatherapy. The air can be filled with soothing aromas from essential oils or incense, which will help you relax even more.
- **Set boundaries**: If you share your space with others, communicate. Let them know that your practice time is sacred, and ask for their support in keeping your environment quiet and undisturbed.
- **Make it personal**: Add elements that are uniquely yours—whether it's a meaningful photograph, an inspiring quote, or a small trinket that keeps you grounded and present.

This space isn't just a corner of your home—it's a reflection of your commitment to honoring yourself, your journey, and your body's wisdom. Create it. Own it. Let it be the place where you reconnect with yourself.

Essential Equipment and Attire

You know the saying: you get what you pay for. Well, that's only true if you're shopping for an expensive watch, not for somatic practice tools. In this world, the "right" equipment isn't about breaking the bank. Nope. It's about simplicity, comfort, and support. Your body doesn't need high-tech gadgets to connect with your inner self—it just needs the basics that allow you to tune in and listen without distractions.

The right gear doesn't need to be flashy, it just needs to do one thing: serve you. Whether that's creating comfort, supporting your movements, or helping you focus—these tools should elevate your experience, not distract from it. And let's not forget about your attire—because if your clothes are too tight or too stiff, your mind will be stuck focusing on the discomfort. This is somatic practice, not a fashion runway. Your clothes should move with you, let you breathe, and, most importantly, allow you to feel every shift and breath your body takes.

Essential Equipment and Attire for Somatic Practice

1. **Comfortable Mat:** A yoga or exercise mat is a non-negotiable. It provides cushioning and helps define your practice space. Go for a mat that's thick enough to support you but firm enough to keep you grounded. You don't want to feel like you're sinking into a marshmallow, but you also don't want to end up on a hard floor. Find your sweet spot.

2. **Loose, Breathable Clothing:** You're not doing your body any favors by cramming it into restrictive fabrics. Go for clothes that breathe, move with you, and don't make you feel like you're in a straightjacket. Think:

SOMATIC EXERCISES FOR NERVOUS SYSTEM REGULATION

- Loose-fitting T-shirts or tank tops
- Comfortable pants or shorts
- Stretchy leggings that feel like second skin

3. **Blanket or Throw:** For those moments when you need extra warmth or padding. It's like a cozy hug for your body during floor exercises.

4. **Pillows or Bolsters:** These bad boys are key for keeping your body aligned and comfortable during different exercises. Support where you need it, when you need it.

5. **Small Towel:** Sweat happens, especially in more active practices. Keep a towel nearby to wipe away the evidence, or use it for extra cushion when your mat just isn't cutting it.

6. **Water Bottle:** You need to stay hydrated to keep your muscles happy and your mind focused. Don't let dehydration interrupt your flow.

7. **Journal and Pen:** After your practice, write it all down. Your body will send you a million messages, and if you don't catch them, they'll slip away. Document your sensations, insights, or progress. You'll thank yourself later.

8. **Timer or Clock:** Timing matters. Use a timer (not your phone—don't get sucked into your email) to track your sessions. Stay present without needing to check the clock every five minutes.

9. **Foam Roller:** This is for those of you who like to go the extra mile. A foam roller is an amazing tool for self-massage and loosening up tight muscles. Totally optional, but oh-so-worth it.

10. **Therapy Balls:** Tennis balls aren't just for playing fetch. Use them to target those stubborn spots that need a little extra pressure and release.

11. **Eye Pillow:** For those blissful moments when you just want to shut out the world and get into the zone. Perfect for relaxation exercises or anytime you're lying down.

12. **Socks or Warm Footwear:** When you're doing those less active exercises, keeping your feet warm can make a huge difference. No one wants to be thinking about cold toes during a moment of calm.

You don't need everything on this list to begin your practice. Start simple—comfortable clothing, a mat, and an open mind. As you grow, you'll discover what works best for your body, and you can slowly add to your toolkit. Your practice is unique to you. Embrace the essentials, and let the rest come in time.

Recommendations for Selecting Yoga Mats and Props

Now that you're equipped with the essentials, let's talk about how to pick the right gear for somatic practice. Your equipment doesn't need to be fancy, but it should be functional and comfortable. Here's what to look for:

Yoga Mats

1. **Thickness:** For somatic work, a mat between 4-6mm thick is your sweet spot. Not too soft that you feel like you're sinking into it, but just thick enough to provide support during floor exercises. It's like the Goldilocks of mats—just right.
2. **Material:** Go eco-friendly, my friend. Look for mats made from natural rubber, cork, or jute. They'll give you that perfect grip, plus they're better for the planet.
3. **Texture:** A textured surface gives you better grip, especially if you sweat like you're training for a marathon. Slip-resistant is key because, let's face it, nobody wants to end up in an unplanned splits moment.
4. **Size:** Standard mats are usually 68" x 24"—that's the size that works for most people. But if you're tall and love to stretch out, go for a longer mat (72" or 74"). No need to feel cramped.
5. **Durability:** Buy once, cry once. A quality mat will last. Brands like Manduka, Jade, and Lululemon have built reputations for durability—so you're not replacing your mat every six months.

Your somatic practice is about you. It's about building a space and selecting tools that honor your body's needs. Your gear should work for you, not the other way around. Get comfortable, get mindful, and let the magic unfold.

Props

When it comes to props, think of them as tools for building your ideal somatic practice—not decorations. If you can, test out the equipment before purchasing. Many yoga and wellness stores let you try out mats and props. That hands-on experience is invaluable because, let's face it, the perfect mat for your body might feel like a piece of junk to someone else. Find the props that work for you. Don't just buy something because it's trendy—get the gear that complements your practice and body.

- **Bolsters**
    - **Firmness:** Look for a firm bolster, at least 24" long. It should provide solid support for your body so you don't feel like you're sinking into it.
    - **Removable Covers:** If you're going to be using your bolster regularly, get

one with a removable, washable cover. Trust me, your future self will thank you when it's time for a cleaning.

- **Blankets**
  - **Mexican Yoga Blankets**: These are solid, sturdy, and versatile. They give you the perfect mix of comfort and support, and they're a classic.
  - **Material:** Opt for 100% cotton. It's breathable, easy to care for, and it won't trap heat in the middle of your practice.

- **Blocks**
  - **Cork Blocks:** For the eco-conscious, cork blocks are sturdy, eco-friendly, and provide excellent support.
  - **Foam Blocks:** Want something softer and lighter? Go for high-density foam blocks. They're comfortable and lightweight without sacrificing support.

- **Straps**
  - **Cotton Straps:** Cotton straps with a D-ring or quick-release buckle are easy to adjust and provide great support for stretching and deepening your poses.
  - **Length:** Go for an 8-10 foot strap. That gives you enough versatility for a variety of poses and practices.

- **Meditation Cushions**
  - **Firmness:** Choose a cushion that's filled with buckwheat hulls. It provides great stability and won't shift under you during seated meditation or practices.
  - **Washable Cover:** Always check that the cover is removable and washable. That's just basic hygiene, folks.

- **Therapy Balls**
  - **Variety Pack**: Start with a set that has multiple sizes—think tennis, lacrosse, and softball-sized balls. Each size offers different types of pressure and release.
  - **Density:** Different densities = different levels of pressure. Pick balls with varying firmness to customize your therapy sessions based on the areas you're targeting.

CHAPTER 2: GETTING STARTED WITH SOMATIC EXERCISES

Tips for Choosing Comfortable Clothing for Somatic Practice

The right clothing is like a second skin. It shouldn't distract you or get in your way—because when you're in the middle of your somatic practice, the last thing you want to worry about is your outfit. Here's how to choose the best gear to enhance your experience:

Prioritize Comfort

Pick clothes that feel good on your body. If something digs into your skin or restricts your movement, get rid of it. You're here to move freely, not to fight with your clothing.

Opt for Breathable Fabrics

Natural fibers like cotton and bamboo are great. They breathe well and keep you cool. If you're into moisture-wicking fabrics, look for those, but avoid anything that feels suffocating or too clingy.

- **Fit Is Key**
    - **Tops:** You want tops that let your arms move freely, but they shouldn't be so loose that they fall over your face during inversions.
    - **Bottoms:** Your legs need freedom. Find bottoms that stretch and move with you without slipping or bunching up.
- **Consider Layering:** Wear layers you can easily add or shed. As you move through different stages of your practice, your body temperature will change. Layers let you adjust on the fly.
- **Avoid Distractions:** Zippers, buttons, scratchy tags—no, no, and no. These little things can cause major discomfort when you're trying to focus. Also, avoid overly loose clothing that might get in the way, like drawstrings or overly baggy pants.
- **Coverage:** You want clothing that makes you feel secure. If you're worried about your clothes shifting or falling out of place, it'll be hard to relax into your practice. Look for things that stay put.
- **Don't Forget Your Feet:** Bare feet are common in somatic practices, but if it's chilly or you're in a relaxation period, have socks on hand. They'll keep your feet cozy and prevent distraction.
- **Consider the Waistband:** Find bottoms with a wide, comfortable waistband. You don't want something digging into your abdomen while you're bending or twisting. Comfort is key.

- **Test for Opacity:** If you're rocking leggings or fitted pants, test them out in front of a mirror. You don't want to risk an accidental wardrobe malfunction when you're reaching for a stretch.
- **Keep It Simple:** You don't need fancy, high-end workout clothes. The basics from your existing wardrobe often work just fine—just make sure they're comfortable, breathable, and flexible.

Ultimately, your clothes should help you forget about them and focus on your body. When your clothing works with you instead of against you, that's when your somatic practice reaches its full potential. It might take a little experimenting, but trust your body to let you know what feels right.

Setting Realistic Goals

Ah, the enthusiasm, ambition, and sometimes a bit too much pressure that come with beginning something new. It's alluring! However, to believe that you'll become a yoga guru or somatic master overnight is only going to lead to disillusionment and exhaustion.

When we don't see drastic results instantly, we start thinking we're not good enough or the practice isn't for us. But here's the kicker: somatic exercise isn't about the dramatic "before and after" shots—it's about subtle, gradual shifts that take time to truly manifest. You've got to honor the process.

Like growing a plant, somatic work takes time to develop but eventually becomes stronger and more rooted in the land (or, in this case, your body). Nevertheless, the secret to maintaining motivation without burning out is to set reasonable, attainable goals. So, let's focus on goals that honor the quiet, beautiful nature of somatic practice.

- **Consistency Over Intensity:** Instead of aiming for marathon-length sessions, aim for 10-15 minutes daily. Little, consistent bursts of somatic work add up, and this will keep you coming back for more without the pressure of big, exhausting sessions.
- **Body Awareness:** Challenge yourself to notice three new sensations in your body each week during your practice. Somatic work is about noticing the subtleties, so focusing on new feelings every week sharpens your awareness and connection.
- **Stress Reduction:** Choose one simple somatic technique—whether it's conscious breathing or progressive muscle relaxation—and aim to do it once a day when stress arises. No need to reinvent the wheel; even the simplest techniques can be powerful tools to manage stress over time.
- **Improved Sleep:** Incorporate a short somatic routine into your bedtime ritual

CHAPTER 2: GETTING STARTED WITH SOMATIC EXERCISES

three nights a week. If sleep is a struggle, somatic work can help calm the body and mind, prepping you for a better night's rest. It doesn't need to be long—just enough to signal your body that it's time to unwind.

- **Pain Management:** If you've got chronic pain, set a goal to reduce it by one point on a 1-10 scale for a month. Regular practice can help manage pain gently and effectively without the pressure of instant results.

- **Mindfulness:** Each time you practice, challenge yourself to stay present and focused for one minute longer than the session before. It's not about perfection; it's about expanding your capacity for mindfulness with each practice.

- **Emotional Regulation:** Try to identify and name one emotion you feel in your body during each session. Somatic work isn't just about physical movement—it's about reconnecting with the emotional landscape of your body. Naming emotions can help you process and release them instead of holding onto them.

- **Flexibility:** Rather than trying to touch your toes in a week, focus on feeling a slight increase in ease of movement in a particular area—like your shoulders or hips—by the end of the month. Somatic work is about fluidity and ease, not extreme flexibility.

- **Self-Compassion:** When discomfort or limitations arise, practice responding with kindness instead of frustration. Treat your body as you would a friend—no judgment, just compassion. This shift in mindset can do wonders for your practice.

- **Integration:** Pick one principle from your somatic practice—like mindful breathing or body scanning—and apply it to a daily activity once a week. Integration is about blending your practice into real life, so it doesn't just stay on the mat—it becomes part of who you are.

By setting goals that are focused on consistency, awareness, and small but meaningful changes, you honor the true spirit of somatic work. Remember, it's a marathon, not a sprint, and every small step forward counts.

Chapter 3: The Forms of Somatic Exercises

To keep the body in good health is a duty... otherwise, we shall not be able to keep our mind strong and clear—Buddha

After a heart-pounding run, sweat is pouring down your cheeks like a medal of honor. Your heart is racing, your muscles are buzzing, and you're almost tingling from the afterglow of success.

Then, after conducting a gentle stretch or a tranquil meditation, picture yourself floating in a sea of serenity, centered, grounded, and at peace. Your body can transition between dialects with ease, opening up a whole new universe of feelings and advantages. It's like your body is a master linguist.

Somatic exercises are no different. These practices are like speaking a new language with your body—each one delivering a different "message," dialing into different sensations and states of being. Some will ground you, making you feel like your roots are sinking deep into the earth, solid and unshakable. Others? They'll lift you up, like a weight you never knew you were carrying is suddenly gone—light, free, and unburdened.

In this chapter, think of these somatic exercises as a tasting menu for your body and mind. We're going to sample a bit of everything, a buffet of movements and sensations. You'll find what resonates, what clicks—whether it's slow, deliberate movements that make you feel deeply connected to yourself or the rhythmic, flowing movements that light up your spirit. You'll find your perfect flavor, your perfect groove.

The History of Somatic Exercise

Somatic exercise doesn't just appear—it's got roots that stretch back over a century, winding through the realms of dance, psychology, and that mind-body connection we're always chasing. Now, the word "somatics" wasn't really thrown around until the 1970s, but the core principles had been quietly brewing in the background long before that, like a pot of coffee waiting to be served.

F.M. Alexander, back in the 1890s, was one of the first pioneers in this field. A struggling actor, plagued by chronic voice loss, Alexander had a lightbulb moment—he realized that his posture and movement patterns were the source of his issues. So, he dug in and started examining how the way he moved through the world was wrecking his voice. What he uncovered laid the groundwork for understanding how those ingrained tension patterns can affect your entire existence. No big deal, right? Just changing how you move can change your life.

Then, along came Moshe Feldenkrais in the 1920s and 30s. A physicist and judo practitioner, Feldenkrais took his debilitating knee injury as an invitation to dig deep into how we move. And boom—out came a system of gentle, precise movements designed to improve both the body and the mind. No biggie—just reshaping physical and mental functioning with a little science and a whole lot of body awareness.

At the same time, dancers like Mabel Elsworth Todd were exploring the relationship between posture, movement, and emotion. She called it "Natural Posture," which later evolved into Ideokinesis—an approach that used mental imagery to shift neuromuscular patterns. Talk about mind over muscle, right?

Fast forward to the 1970s, and bam, enter the term "somatics," thanks to Thomas Hanna. Hanna, influenced by Feldenkrais, developed Hanna Somatic Education, a practice that centers on internal physical perception. Translation? It's all about feeling how you move, not just moving for the sake of it. This was a pivotal moment that catapulted somatic practices into the mainstream.

Later, somatic exercises became popular in physical therapy, psychology, and even conventional medicine, in addition to dance studios and therapy rooms. The ripple effect was enormous. These days, somatic exercise is more than just a specific activity; it's a movement that incorporates every aspect of the mind-body connection and is bound together by the core principle that our emotions are directly influenced by the movements we perform.

How Somatics Work on the Nervous System

Somatic exercises don't just dance around the surface—they go deep, working hand in hand with the nervous system in ways that are nothing short of transformative. They target the sensorimotor system, the very network that governs not only how we move but also how we perceive our body's existence in the vast space around us. Let's break it down and see how this intricate tango between body and brain unfolds:

- **Sensory-Motor Feedback Loop:** Your sensory neurons—those little messengers—send constant updates to your brain about your body's position and movement. Meanwhile, your motor neurons are busy controlling your muscles. Somatic exercises fine-tune this whole feedback loop, creating a beautifully synchronized

CHAPTER 3: THE FORMS OF SOMATIC EXERCISES

conversation between brain and body. By slowing down and moving with intention, you give your nervous system the time it craves to process this feedback with precision, which can lead to a heightened sense of body awareness and control. It's like giving your nervous system the VIP treatment it deserves.

- **Neuroplasticity:** Here's where things get juicy: neuroplasticity. When you repeatedly engage in somatic exercises, you tap into the brain's ability to form new neural connections. Think of it as creating new highways in your brain, smoother and more efficient than the old, bumpy ones. With every mindful movement, you reinforce and solidify these pathways, possibly overriding those stubborn patterns of tension or misalignment you've carried for years. Yes, your brain can rewire itself. Imagine that.

- **Interoception:** Somatic exercises are like turning the volume up on your body's internal radio station—what we call interoception. It's that inner sense, the ability to feel what's happening inside your body. As you practice, you become more attuned to these signals, fine-tuning the feedback from your organs and muscles. This increased awareness can then help regulate the autonomic nervous system, potentially dialing down stress levels and boosting your overall well-being. Your body's whispers become more like an audible conversation.

- **Proprioception:** Have you ever had one of those "Wait, where is my body in space right now?" moments? Somatic practices fine-tune proprioception, your innate sense of where your body is relative to its surroundings. This is your body's internal GPS. The more you work with somatic exercises, the more efficient and accurate this internal navigation becomes, improving your balance, coordination, and the overall ease with which you move. It's like upgrading from a paper map to a GPS navigation system that doesn't need recalculating.

- **Muscular Re-education:** Here's a trick the body's been holding out on you: muscular re-education. Many somatic techniques involve intentionally contracting muscles and then slowly releasing them, a process known as pandiculation. It's like a reset button for your muscles, recalibrating their resting tone and improving how the nervous system governs muscle tension. It's like teaching your muscles to relax again, one gentle movement at a time.

- **Autonomic Nervous System Regulation:** The beauty of somatic exercises is their ability to give the autonomic nervous system (ANS) a nudge—shifting it from the stressed-out, fight-or-flight mode (sympathetic) to the more relaxed, restorative rest-and-digest state (parasympathetic). The slow, mindful nature of these movements allows your nervous system to ease into a state of calm, reducing stress, improving digestion, and making relaxation feel like second nature. It's like having a personal concierge for your nervous system—taking you from chaos to calm in no time.

- **Cortical Remapping:** The brain isn't just some passive observer in the background; it's actively involved in your somatic journey. Focused attention on specific areas of your body during exercises can spark cortical remapping—essentially changing how your brain represents these body parts in the somatosensory cortex. What does that mean for you? Potential pain relief and better motor control. Your brain rewires its map, giving you a sharper, more efficient mental representation of your body. Pain, meet your new roadmap.

- **Vagus Nerve Stimulation:** Some somatic practices, particularly those that involve breath work or gentle movements around the neck and face, have a direct line to your vagus nerve. This mighty nerve plays a crucial role in regulating parasympathetic activity, the part of your nervous system responsible for relaxation and stress resilience. By stimulating this nerve, somatic exercises promote a profound sense of calm, helping you handle stress like a pro. It's like hitting the "reset" button on your stress response, bringing your body back to a state of zen with every breath.

Somatic exercises are more than just physical movements—they're the keys to unlocking a deeper, more harmonious relationship with your nervous system. When your body moves mindfully, everything starts to shift—stress, pain, and tension—all of it starts to melt away, leaving you with nothing but clarity, peace, and a body that truly feels alive.

The Role of the Nervous System in Stress, Anxiety, and Tension

Think of your nervous system as your body's ultimate puppet master, controlling the strings of every single organ. Pulling all the appropriate levers and turning all the dials to keep everything going smoothly—at least most of the time—is what it does as the secret agent and holder of the backstage pass to the thriller that is your life. But what happens when tension, worry, and stress start to creep in? It's as if that agent loses their temper and makes the entire operation into a full-length action film. Let's examine the intricacy and complexity of your nervous system's involvement in all of this.

The Stress Response

The moment stress rears its ugly head—whether it's that "oh crap" deadline looming, a heart-pounding moment in traffic, or that surge of excitement when you've got something big on the horizon—your nervous system doesn't just sit there and watch. Like a military-grade device that has been precisely calibrated to keep you alive, it activates and performs flawlessly.

- **The Amygdala:** The alarm goes off. What does the amygdala do? Serving as your emotional 911 operator. It constantly scans the horizon for dangers, and it sounds the alarm whenever it detects anything even vaguely like danger. This almond-shaped part of your brain doesn't care if it's real or not; if it smells danger, it kicks off the whole show. It tells the hypothalamus, "Get your act together; we need backup!"

- **The HPA Axis Gets in Gear:** Here comes the hormone barrage. The hypothalamus, not skipping a beat, taps into the HPA (hypothalamic-pituitary-adrenal) axis like it's dialing up reinforcements. And voilà—cortisol, the body's favorite stress hormone, surges into your bloodstream. It's like the body's personal version of "Game on!" Getting you ready for action, for whatever chaos is about to unfold.

- **The Sympathetic Nervous System Takes the Wheel:** Boom. This is when your body throws all subtlety out the window. The sympathetic nervous system, that fire-breathing dragon of your autonomic nervous system, flips the "fight-or-flight" switch. Heart rate skyrockets, blood zooms to your muscles like they've been injected with rocket fuel, and your brain sharpens so you can outthink and outmaneuver whatever's coming your way. It's time to perform.

- **Physical Tension Builds:** Tightening muscles? You bet. This is your body's go-to "prepare for war" strategy. Muscles tense, ready to either punch back or sprint away at the first sign of action. Your body's locked and loaded, primed to do whatever it needs to survive.

Anxiety: When the Alarm Gets Stuck

What happens when stress doesn't just pass by but sets up camp? When the body keeps hearing the alarm bells, even when there's no real danger? This is where anxiety steps in, turning your stress-response system into a bad remix that's stuck on a loop. Let's see how your nervous system goes from "I got this" to "Get me off this rollercoaster!"

- **Hypervigilance:** The amygdala, once your reliable alarm system, turns into that crazy security guard who's convinced every leaf is a burglar. It's like your brain just can't turn off the "threat mode," obsessively looking for danger everywhere—even when there's none to be found. The problem? Your mind gets locked in a state of constant alert. You're on edge. All the time. Your brain becomes the poster child for anxiety.

- **Feedback Loop:** This is where the wheels start spinning off. An anxious thought fires up your stress response, which in turn fuels more anxious thoughts, triggering more physical responses. It's like an endless loop, a doom loop where your body is constantly re-triggering the same feelings of fear and panic. There's no off button, no reset. Just the same track, over and over.

- **Autonomic Imbalance:** Your body goes into full-on fight-or-flight mode, but the parasympathetic nervous system—the one that's supposed to help you chill, rest, and recover? It's taking a nap. The sympathetic nervous system stays in control, and it's like your body's been stuck in fast-forward. You're constantly revved up, even though there's no pressing reason to be. Rest? Forget it. Relaxation becomes an afterthought.

- **Neurotransmitter Disruption:** Anxiety doesn't just hijack your body's stress response; it messes with your brain chemistry too. Neurotransmitters like serotonin, GABA, and norepinephrine (the usual suspects in mood regulation) get all scrambled, making it harder to calm down. It's like trying to tune a piano with a broken key. Your mind just isn't in sync, and the cycle continues.

Chronic Tension

When stress and anxiety linger for long enough, the body starts to develop a muscle memory for tension. This isn't the good kind of muscle memory that comes from building strength or learning new movements. This is the "holding-on-for-dear-life" kind. Your body locks in that tension, and bam, it becomes a permanent fixture, like a bad habit you just can't shake off.

- **Muscle Memory:** You don't just forget how to relax. No, no. If you've been perpetually stressed, tensing your muscles without even realizing it, your body gets stuck. It's like being caught in a loop where your muscles stay in "ready-for-action" mode. Even when there's no actual threat, your body stays on high alert, locked in a state of tension, like a coiled spring ready to snap.

- **Pain-Tension Cycle:** Here's the kicker. The more you tense up, the more pain you create. And the more pain you feel, the more your nervous system demands you tighten up. This creates a vicious cycle, like a loop of torment. Tension creates pain, pain creates more tension, and so on. You're stuck in a cage of your own creation.

- **Sensorimotor Amnesia:** Thomas Hanna's brilliant term, sensorimotor amnesia, describes how your brain forgets how to relax muscles that have been tight for so long. It's like your body's turned into a foreign country, and you've completely forgotten the map. Relaxation? Yeah, that's a skill you're going to have to re-learn. Because your body has lost the ability to let go.

The Potential for Relief

The nervous system isn't just a troublemaker; it's also the ultimate peacekeeper, with the potential to rescue you from the jaws of stress, anxiety, and tension. And lucky for you, knowing how it works opens the door to a bunch of potential solutions that can get you out of the stress pit and back to smooth sailing.

- **Vagus Nerve Stimulation:** Think of the vagus nerve as the "off" button for stress. It's the main player in the parasympathetic nervous system—the one that says, "Hey, take a breath, calm down, everything's cool." By activating the vagus nerve, you can shift the body out of "fight-or-flight" and back into "rest-and-digest." You can rewire your system to chill the heck out. How? Try deep breathing, cold showers, or chanting. Yeah, it sounds a little out there, but it works.

- **Interoceptive Awareness:** Here's the deal—your body is trying to tell you when you're stressed. But if you're too busy running around like a chicken with its head cut off, you might miss the memo. Interoceptive awareness is the art of listening to your body's internal signals—your heart rate, breathing, and even muscle tension—and tuning in to them before the stress hits critical levels. It's like learning to read the warning signs before the storm. The earlier you catch it, the easier it is to defuse.

- **Neuroplasticity:** Your brain is like an overzealous electrician constantly rewiring itself. And just like any rewiring job, you can make some serious upgrades. Neuroplasticity is the brain's ability to form new neural connections, which means that even if you've been stuck in the stress loop for ages, you can train your brain to handle it better. Practices like mindfulness, meditation, or somatic exercises can help you reprogram your stress response, turning your mental chaos into calm efficiency.

- **HRV Training:** Heart Rate Variability (HRV) training is like finding the perfect playlist for your nervous system. The more you can sync your heart rate with your breath, the better your body can handle stress. It's all about balancing the autonomic nervous system, that magical duo of your sympathetic (fight-or-flight) and parasympathetic (rest-and-relax) systems.

- **Somatic Exercises:** Your body's been holding onto tension for so long that it's become part of your identity. Somatic exercises help you unlearn that muscle memory, break free from that permanent state of tension, and help your body come back to its natural, relaxed state. These exercises help you reconnect with your body, calm your nervous system, and release chronic tension, leaving you feeling lighter and more in control.

Pioneers of Somatic Exercise: Hanna, Feldenkrais, and Alexander

Now, let's throw it back to the pioneers of somatic exercise—these folks weren't just thinking outside the box; they were flipping the box on its head.

Thomas Hanna: The Name of Somatics Thomas Hanna, a true trailblazer in the world of somatics, didn't just contribute to the field—he named it. He realized that our physical limitations, pains, and chronic tension weren't just part of getting older or some random accident; they were learned habits from poor movement and posture. That's what he called "sensory-motor amnesia"—basically, your body forgetting how to move efficiently.

His method, "Somatic Education," involves slow, deliberate movements that help you regain control over your body. It's like hitting the reset button on your body's operating system. Through focusing on awareness, you unlearn the bad habits that lead to tension and pain. It's all about rediscovering how to move naturally and comfortably again.

But—hold up—here's where people get it wrong. There's a myth that Hanna's work is only about stretching or yoga-type moves. In reality, it's about retraining your body to move in a healthier, more functional way. Think of it as your body's version of a software update. The real deal? It's about breaking the cycle of physical stress, undoing the damage of years of poor movement habits, and using the power of awareness to change your body's relationship with tension.

So, when you're working through somatic exercises, you're not just moving—you're rewriting your body's story, learning how to live and move with more ease.

- **Myth 1:** Hanna Somatics Can Cure All Physical Ailments
  Some enthusiasts claim Hanna Somatics is the holy grail for every physical problem.
- **Reality:** Oh, how we wish it were true. Hanna Somatics is powerful, but it's not some magic pill. While it can do wonders for chronic pain and movement limitations, it's not going to cure everything from a sprained ankle to your existential crisis. It's a tool, not the entire toolbox. So let's not start calling it a panacea, folks. You'll be disappointed, I promise.
- **Myth 2:** Hanna's Work is Just Another Form of Stretching
  Some people think Hanna Somatics is just stretching with a fancy name.
- **Reality:** Nice try. Stretching and Hanna Somatics are like comparing a cardboard box to a luxury car. Stretching is just pulling on your muscles; Hanna Somatics

CHAPTER 3: THE FORMS OF SOMATIC EXERCISES

is about rewiring your brain to control your muscles better. We're talking pandiculation, which is a mix of gentle contraction and slow, mindful release. It's all about resetting your muscle tone and fixing your brain's control system. Stretching can't do that. Sorry, no shortcuts here.

- **Myth 3:** Somatic Exercises Are Only for the Elderly or Those in Pain
  Some people think Hanna Somatics is only for the elderly or people in chronic pain.

- **Reality:** That's like saying yoga is only for the flexible. Yes, Hanna Somatics is great for those dealing with pain or getting on in years, but it's also a goldmine for athletes, office workers, and even kids. It's about improving movement and body awareness—everybody's got muscles, folks, and they can all benefit. Everyone deserves smoother, more efficient movement.

- **Myth 4:** Hanna Claimed to Have Invented Somatics
  Some people think Hanna invented the whole field of somatics.

- **Reality:** Close, but no cigar. While Hanna coined the term and expanded the field, he wasn't the sole creator. He recognized and respected the contributions of others like Feldenkrais and even credited them as his influences. He was part of a bigger movement—he didn't just pop up out of nowhere with all the answers. He built on what came before him. Collaboration, people, collaboration.

- **Myth 5:** Hanna Somatics Requires No Effort
  There's a belief that because Hanna Somatics is gentle, it doesn't require effort.

- **Reality:** Just because you're not breaking a sweat doesn't mean you're not working. Hanna Somatics may not leave you gasping for air, but it sure demands mental effort. It's about focusing, paying attention, and being patient with your body. If you think you're going to experience magic without putting in the effort, you're in for a rude awakening. Regular practice, mental discipline, and commitment—that's where the change happens.

- **Myth 6:** Hanna's Ideas Aren't Scientifically Supported
  Some naysayers argue that Hanna's methods lack scientific backing.

- **Reality:** Cue the eye roll. When Hanna first came up with this stuff, sure, there wasn't much scientific proof to back it up. But guess what? Times have changed. Now, the core principles like neuroplasticity (the brain's ability to change and adapt) are backed by neuroscience. So it's not just some fluffy idea floating in the ether anymore. The research is catching up—finally.

Moshe Feldenkrais: The Physicist of Movement

Moshe Feldenkrais (1904–1984) was a true Renaissance man: a physicist, engineer, martial artist, and movement pioneer. After suffering a debilitating knee injury, he applied his analytical mind to the problem of human movement and healing. He developed two complementary methods: Functional Integration (hands-on, one-on-one sessions) and Awareness Through Movement (verbally guided group classes). Both aim to improve movement and function by increasing body awareness and exploring new movement patterns.

Feldenkrais's approach is all about learning—not exercising or correcting. He believed that if you give the nervous system better information, it will naturally choose more efficient, comfortable ways of moving—like upgrading your body's software by expanding its movement vocabulary.

F.M. Alexander: The Posture Pioneer

Frederick Matthias Alexander (1869–1955) was an Australian actor who developed vocal problems that threatened his career. Alexander discovered that his vocal issues were linked to his overall posture and the way he held tension in his body. He developed a technique to consciously improve posture and reduce unnecessary tension, particularly in the head, neck, and back.

The Alexander Technique, as it came to be known, is about becoming aware of habitual ways of holding and moving your body that may be causing pain or limiting your function. It's like learning to read the user manual for your own body, understanding how your thoughts and intentions translate into physical actions.

The Common Thread

While Hanna, Feldenkrais, and Alexander developed distinct methods, they share common principles:

- **Mindfulness:** All three emphasize the importance of paying attention to what you're doing with your body.
- **Neuroplasticity:** They recognized, before it was scientifically proven, that the brain can change and that movement patterns can be relearned.
- **Holistic Approach:** Each saw the body and mind as an interconnected whole, not separate entities.
- **Gentle Exploration:** Rather than forceful exercise, they advocated for gentle, mindful movement to create change.
- **Empowerment:** All three methods aim to give people tools to help themselves rather than relying solely on a practitioner.

CHAPTER 3: THE FORMS OF SOMATIC EXERCISES

Some questions have been stirring lately: How much joy can a nervous system hold? How much pleasure can it contain? How much kindness can it embrace? How much slowness can it savor?

I am learning that we can gradually expand our capacity for stillness, slowness, and softness because the nervous system is a living, breathing entity—one that can expand, soften, and grow. With each breath, each mindful movement, the boundaries of bodily experience stretch ever so slightly, gently coaxing the body to open up, to let in more of life's richness.

Chapter 4: Managing Anxiety with Somatic Exercise

In the rhythm of movement, anxiety loses its grip; each breath, each step, a return to calm.

Ever heard that anxiety is just your brain time-traveling to every worst-case scenario imaginable? That hit me hard. Why couldn't I just stop worrying like everyone said? For the longest time, I thought I was broken. Turns out my body wasn't the enemy—it was trying to help me all along.

The game-changer? One tiny shift. Whenever I feel that creeping unease, I place my hand on my chest. Simple, right? But it's like hitting the emergency brakes on my nervous system. As I feel my heartbeat beneath my palm, I remind myself: Uncertainty is where possibility lives. Uncertainty is where freedom lives.

At first, it felt ridiculous. How could embracing uncertainty make me feel safe? But as I practiced, something clicked. That small gesture built a bridge between my runaway thoughts and my body's sensations. It pulled me back to right now, where anxiety doesn't stand a chance.

I started recognizing anxiety's telltale signs—the tight chest, the shallow breaths, the clenched jaw. But instead of spiraling, I saw them as signals: Pause. Breathe. Come back. This little ritual didn't erase my anxiety overnight, but it gave me something better—a way to anchor myself when the storm hits. I've learned to trust my body's wisdom instead of fighting it.

Understanding Anxiety and Its Triggers

Do you know what used to send my anxiety through the roof? Grocery stores. Yeah, grocery stores. The fluorescent lights, the endless aisles, the existential crisis over choosing between 15 kinds of peanut butter—it all conspired against me. More than once, I left a full cart in the middle of the store and bolted for the exit. My brain knew it wasn't rational, but anxiety doesn't do logic.

What I didn't realize then was that my body was sending up flares: Hey, something doesn't feel safe here. It wasn't the groceries—it was a trigger. A place where past stress and future dread collided, and my nervous system decided to sound the alarm.

Anxiety is a tangled mess of body and mind. Biologically, it's our ancient survival system kicking in. Your amygdala (the brain's built-in security guard) senses a threat—real or imagined—and fires off distress signals. Adrenaline and cortisol flood your system. Your heart races, breathing gets shallow, and muscles tense. If you were facing a bear, this would be useful. But when the 'threat' is a social gathering or a tough decision? Not so much.

Psychologically, anxiety hijacks your thoughts. It feeds on worst-case scenarios, loops intrusive worries, and convinces you that disaster is imminent. Then, your racing mind tells your racing heart, Yep, something must be wrong!—and the cycle repeats. Breaking free means addressing both mind and body, which is why somatic techniques work so well.

Anxiety isn't one-size-fits-all, but here are some usual suspects:

1. **Social situations:** Crowds, strangers, or just making small talk can send some people into full-blown panic mode.
2. **Performance pressure:** Work presentations, exams, or anything where you're being judged? Cue the sweaty palms.
3. **Health concerns:** Your own health or a loved one's, especially during uncertain times, can be a major trigger.
4. **Financial stress:** Money worries, job security, big purchases—nothing like finances to spike cortisol levels.
5. **Major life changes:** Even good changes (new job, marriage, moving) come with uncertainty, which anxiety loves.
6. **Conflict:** Whether it's a full-blown argument or just an awkward conversation, tension can be a major trigger.
7. **Phobias:** Heights, tight spaces, certain animals—specific fears can trigger intense anxiety responses.
8. **Trauma reminders:** Sounds, smells, or situations linked to past trauma can send your nervous system into overdrive.
9. **Decision-making:** Some people freeze up over any decision, big or small.
10. **Lack of control:** Feeling powerless in a situation is anxiety's favorite playground.

Understanding these triggers is the first step. The next? Learning how to navigate them without getting swept away.

Somatic Movement for Anxiety Relief

Before you start working through the exercises, remember that you can scan the QR code at the beginning of the book for a more detailed, visual interpretation of the exercises. May your journey be restorative, healing, soothing, and incredibly rewarding!

Here is the QR code again as a quick reminder.

https://aredpen.com/sen

The body loves movement. It craves it, thrives on it, and uses it as a language to communicate with us. When we engage in mindful, intentional movements, we create a dialogue with our body; we give it a chance to express itself, release pent-up tension, and find its way back to balance. Somatic movements for anxiety relief invite you to tune in, listen attentively, and allow your body to guide you toward a state of calm. In this section, we'll explore how simple movements can become powerful tools for managing anxiety, helping you not just cope with stress but move through it with grace and resilience.

Cat-Cow Pose (Marjaryasana-Bitilasana)

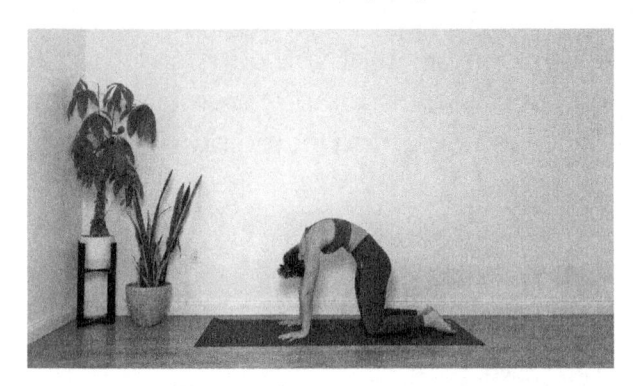

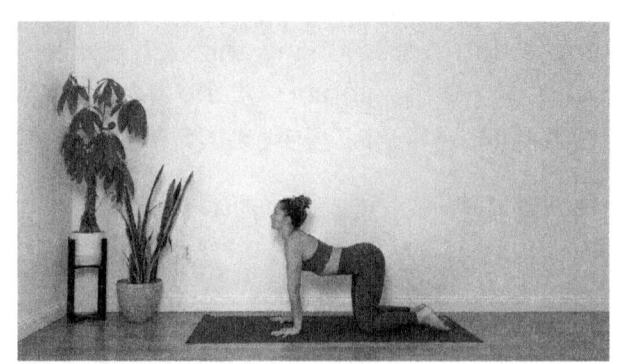

This simple yet powerful yoga flow loosens up your spine, shakes the tension out of your shoulders and neck, and gets your breath and body working together like old friends.

1. **Cat Pose (Exhale):** Round your spine toward the ceiling like a stretching cat who just woke up from a nap. Tuck your chin, scoop your belly in, and let everything curl inward—like you're bracing for drama but staying composed.

2. **Cow Pose (Inhale):** Flip the script. Arch your back, lift your chest and tailbone skyward, and let your belly melt toward the floor. Gaze up slightly, like you just remembered something delightful.

3. Keep this movement flowing—exhale for Cat, inhale for Cow—letting your breath be the DJ, setting the pace.

4. Repeat 5-10 cycles, moving slow and smooth, like you're pouring honey over tight spots and letting stiffness dissolve.

Dynamic Child's Pose (Balasana) with Arm Reaches

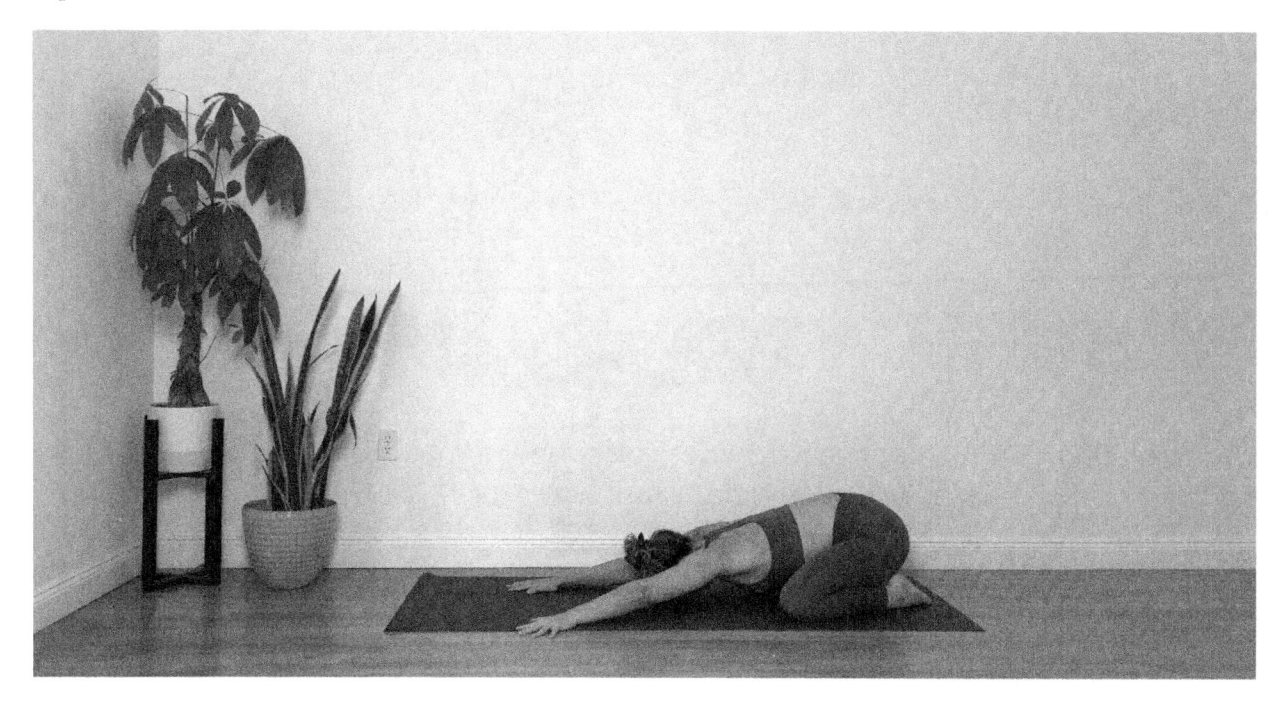

This is a variation of the traditional Child's Pose that incorporates arm movements. It helps release tension in the back, shoulders, and hips while promoting a sense of grounding and safety.

1. Start in a kneeling position, then sit back on your heels.
2. Fold forward, lowering your chest toward your thighs and extending your arms out in front of you.
3. Take a few deep breaths here, feeling the stretch in your back.
4. As you inhale, sweep your right arm up and to the right, creating a half-circle motion.
5. Exhale as you bring the arm back down to the starting position.
6. Repeat with the left arm.
7. Continue alternating arms for 5-10 cycles on each side, moving slowly and breathing deeply.

SOMATIC EXERCISES FOR NERVOUS SYSTEM REGULATION

Spinal Rolls (Seated or Standing)

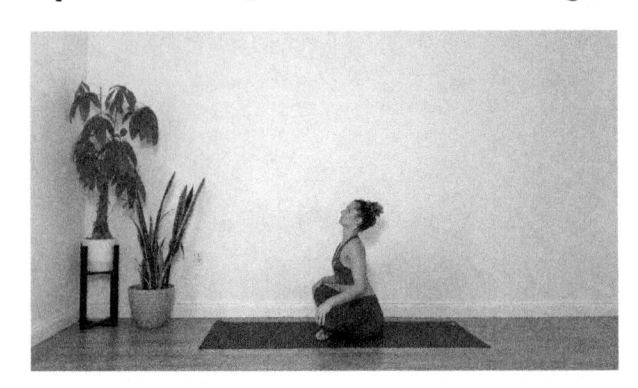

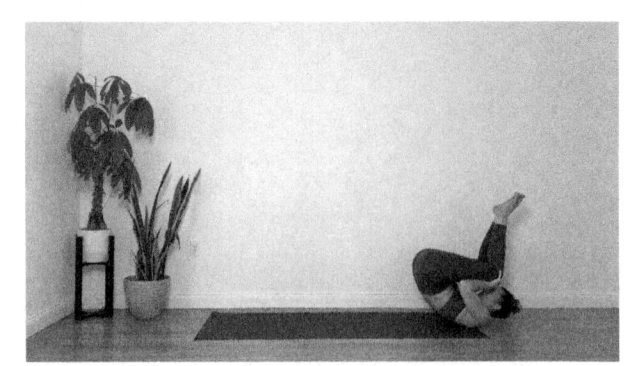

Our spine carries the weight of our modern disconnect. These rolls help reestablish the communication between mind and body that we've lost in our hurried lives.

1. Sit on the floor with your legs crossed in a comfortable position for your body.
2. Place your hands on your knees as anchors for stability.
3. Inhale as you lift your chest and slightly arch your back, creating space where tension usually dominates.
4. Exhale while rounding your spine, bringing your chin toward your chest and navel toward your spine.
5. Continue this mindful rolling motion, using your breath as your guide rather than rushing through.
6. Complete 5-10 cycles, noticing how your body begins to remember its natural wisdom.

Steps for Standing Spinal Rolls:

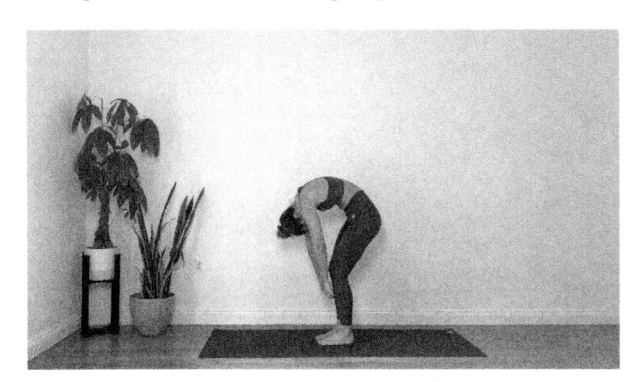

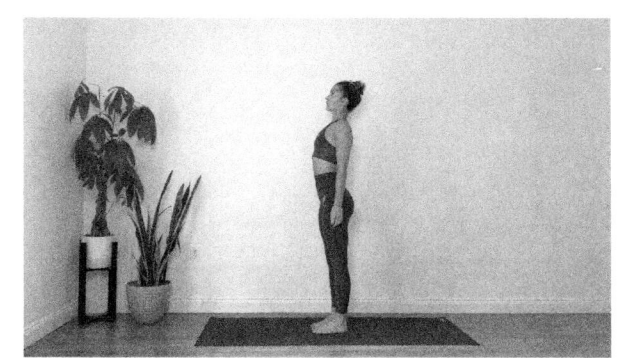

1. Stand with feet hip-width apart, knees slightly bent to support your lower back.

2. As you inhale, roll your shoulders back, lift your chest, and look up—countering the forward slump of desk work.

3. With your exhale, round forward, tucking chin and reaching arms ahead, releasing the day's accumulated stress.

4. Allow this rolling movement to continue with deliberate awareness rather than mechanical repetition.

5. Your arms should hang naturally, moving in response to your spine rather than through forced effort.

6. Repeat for 5-10 cycles, each one an opportunity to reconnect with the body you've been too busy to listen to.

SOMATIC EXERCISES FOR NERVOUS SYSTEM REGULATION

Pelvic Tilts

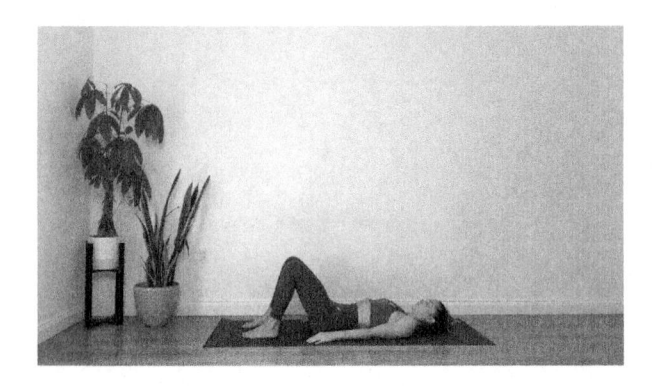

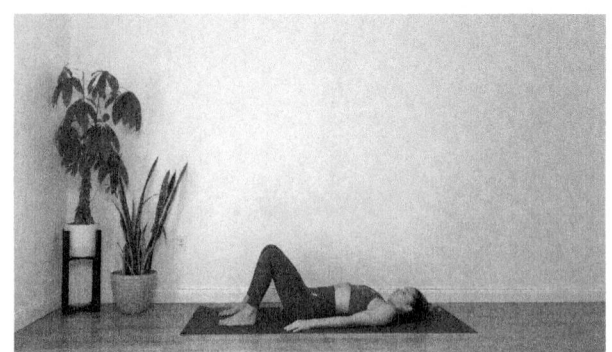

Your pelvis—the bowl that cradles your center—often bears the burden of modern disconnection. This gentle rocking motion isn't just exercise; it's a conversation with your foundation, an invitation to release what your lower back has been holding.

1. Rest your body on its back, knees bent like bridges, feet grounded hip-width apart.
2. Allow your arms to surrender beside you, palms connecting with the earth.
3. Draw breath in, belly rising like the tide—a natural wisdom your body remembers.
4. As you exhale, tilt your pelvis upward in a gentle nod, pressing your spine into the floor. Feel how your abdomen awakens to this dialogue.
5. With your next inhale, return to neutral, allowing the natural curve of your lower back to reclaim its space.
6. Continue this mindful rhythm for 10-15 cycles.

Gentle Neck Rolls

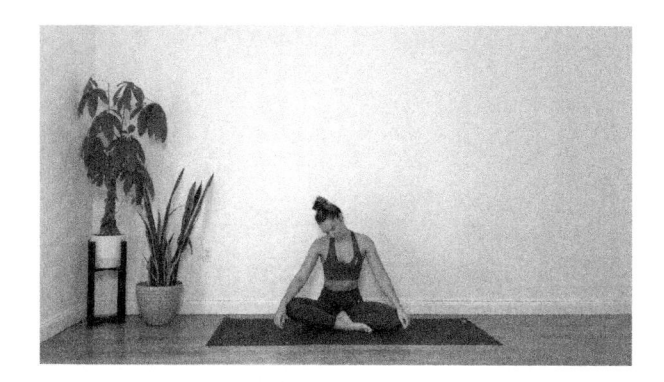

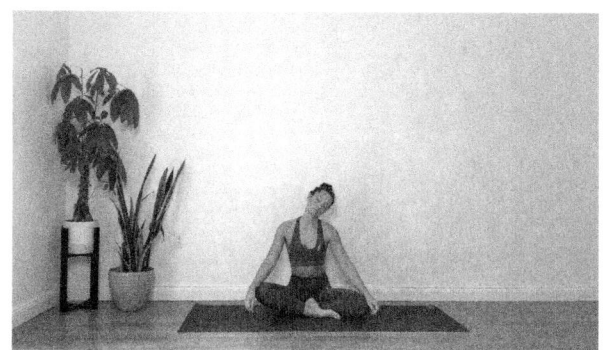

The neck—a pillar between thought and action—carries the weight of decisions unmade and tensions unaddressed. These rolls aren't merely stretches; they're a release of the stories your shoulders have been silently telling.

1. Find yourself seated with dignity, spine rising like a mountain, whether on the floor or in a chair.
2. Allow your chin to bow forward, honoring the stretch that awakens across your neck's back terrain.
3. With intention, roll your awareness rightward, right ear drawing toward welcoming shoulder.
4. Continue this journey upward, gaze meeting the sky in quiet acknowledgment.
5. Complete your circle by visiting the left ear and shoulder in momentary communion before returning home.
6. Trace this path 3-5 times, then reverse the pilgrimage for another 3-5 cycles.

Constructive Rest Position

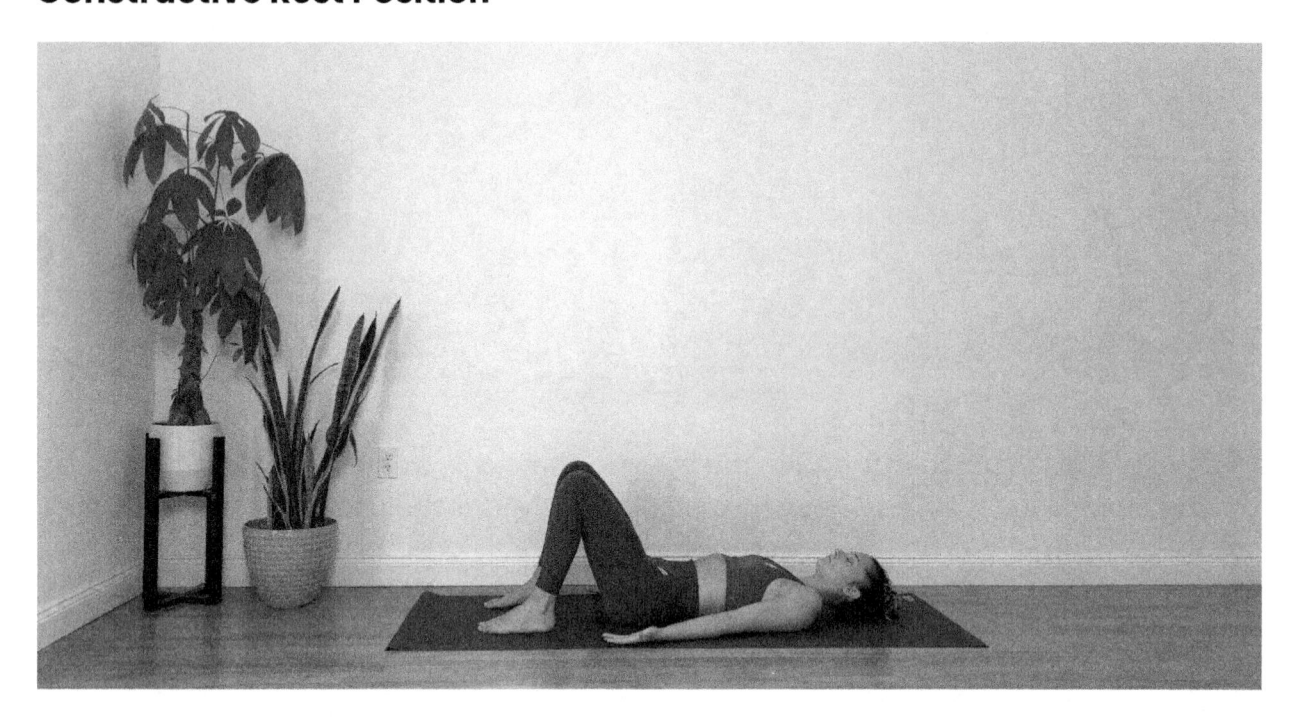

In a world that demands constant doing, this position offers the radical alternative of being. It's not laziness but a return to the body's forgotten intelligence—a reset for the nervous system that's been running on emergency power for too long.

1. Lay your body on flat ground, surrendering to gravity.
2. Bend your knees skyward, feet planted firmly at hip's width.
3. Let your arms rest beside you, palms open to receive what's been waiting for your attention.
4. Shield your eyes from distraction, bringing awareness to the breath that's been with you all along.
5. Listen for the stories of tension in your body, granting permission for their release.
6. Remain in this dialogue for 5-15 minutes

Arch and Flatten

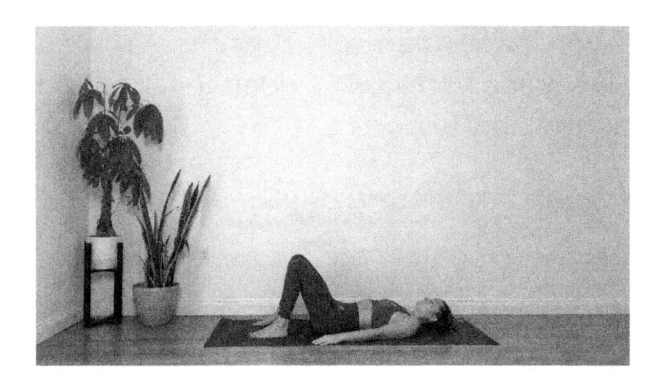

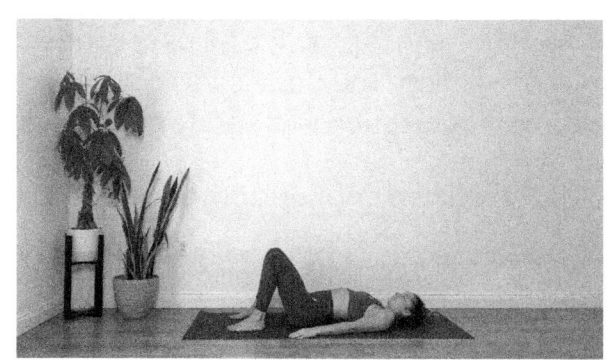

The lower spine—a curved bridge between earth and sky—speaks volumes about our relationship with stability. This rhythmic motion isn't just movement; it's relearning the language of your core, the foundation you've built walls around in the rush of modern life.

1. Find rest on your back, knees bent in preparation, feet establishing connection at hip's width.
2. Allow arms to settle beside you, palms receiving the ground's support.
3. As breath enters, allow your lower back to arch gently—a small act of courage creating space where compression has ruled.
4. With exhale's wisdom, press your spine earthward, awakening the abdominal center that modern life has silenced.
5. Continue this sacred conversation—inhale to open, exhale to ground.
6. Repeat this, remembering for 10-15 cycles, each motion guided by the natural rhythm.

SOMATIC EXERCISES FOR NERVOUS SYSTEM REGULATION

Body Scan

This mindfulness practice helps reconnect with your body when daily stress has created disconnection. The body scan helps increase awareness, release hidden tension, and promote relaxation that many of us have forgotten how to access.

1. Lie down comfortably on your back with your arms resting at your sides.
2. Close your eyes and take a few deep breaths to center your awareness.
3. Begin by focusing on your toes. Notice any sensations present without trying to change them.
4. Gradually move your attention upward through your feet, ankles, and legs, paying attention to what you find.
5. At each body part, pause momentarily. Notice what sensations, tensions, or emotions might be stored there.
6. When you discover areas of tension, imagine breathing directly into that spot, allowing natural release.
7. Continue this systematic awareness through your entire body.
8. Finish with several conscious breaths before gently returning to your surroundings. This practice takes between 5 and 30 minutes, depending on how thoroughly you explore each area.

Progressive Muscle Relaxation

Many of us have forgotten how to recognize tension in our bodies, carrying it unknowingly throughout our day. PMR teaches the difference between tension and relaxation by creating deliberate contrast—helping you rediscover what letting go feels like.

1. Find a comfortable position, either sitting or lying down.
2. Start with your feet. Deliberately tense the muscles for 5 seconds.
3. Release completely, paying attention to the sensation of relief for 10-15 seconds.
4. Move up to your calves. Create tension here for 5 seconds, then release.
5. Continue this pattern upward: thighs, buttocks, abdomen, chest, arms, hands, shoulders, neck, and face.
6. For each muscle group, maintain tension for 5 seconds, followed by 10-15 seconds of conscious release.
7. Notice the difference between these states in each area of your body.

8. After completing the full sequence, take several deep breaths and observe how your body feels.

Grounding Techniques

When anxiety pulls us out of our bodies, these practices serve as anchors to the present moment. They're practical tools for returning awareness from scattered thoughts to physical reality.

5-4-3-2-1 Technique:

1. Find a supportive seated position.
2. Take several centering breaths.
3. Connect with your surroundings by noting:

    - 5 things you can see
    - 4 things you can touch
    - 3 things you can hear
    - 2 things you can smell
    - 1 thing you can taste

- Give each sense your full attention, noticing details you might normally miss.

Physical Grounding:

1. Stand barefoot, preferably on natural ground.
2. Focus on the sensation where your feet meet the earth.
3. Imagine roots extending downward from your feet, creating stability.
4. Breathe deeply, visualizing supportive energy rising from the ground into your body.
5. Continue for 5-10 minutes, until you feel more centered and present.

SOMATIC EXERCISES FOR NERVOUS SYSTEM REGULATION

Somatic Twists

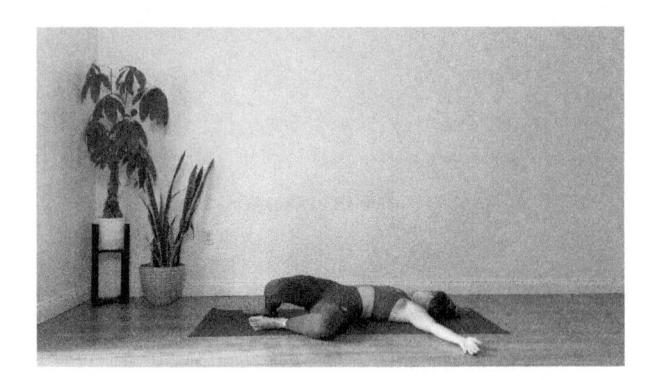

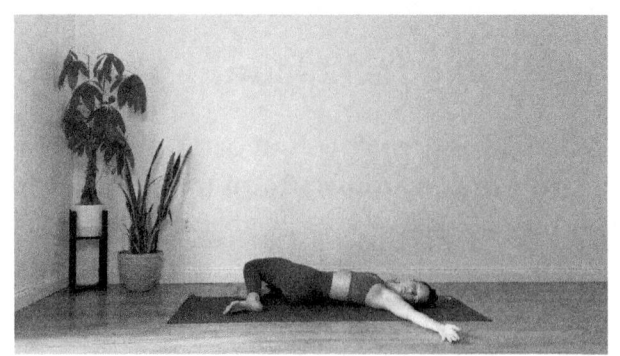

The spine often holds tension from daily stress and worry. These gentle rotations help release tightness in your back and promote mobility that anxiety tends to restrict.

1. Lie on your back with knees bent, feet flat on the floor at hip-width.
2. Extend your arms outward in a T-position for stability.
3. Keeping shoulders grounded, allow both knees to fall gently to the right.
4. Turn your head left, creating a gentle twist through your spine.
5. Hold for 5-10 complete breaths, feeling the gradual release.
6. Mindfully return knees and head to center.
7. Repeat on the opposite side, knees left and head right.
8. Complete 3-5 repetitions on each side, moving with deliberate awareness.

Tabletop Arm and Leg Extensions

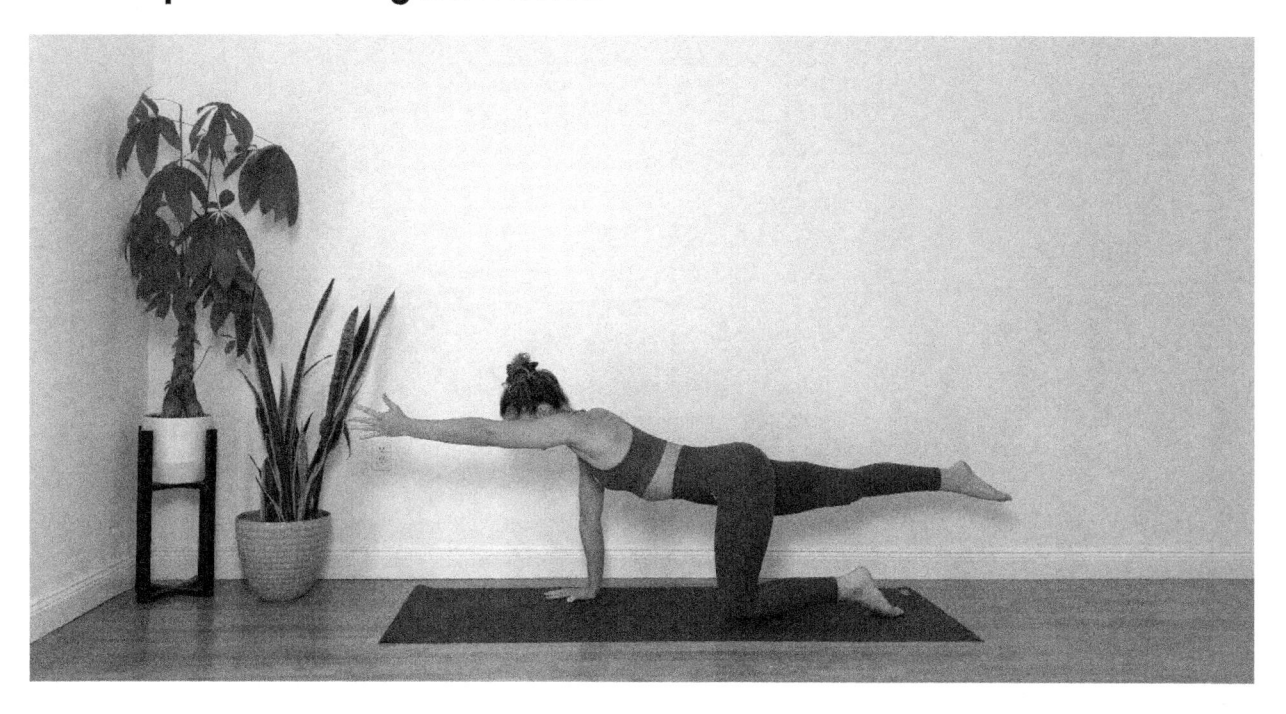

This balanced movement requires focus that anxiety often disrupts. By coordinating opposite limbs while stabilizing your core, you practice the centered attention that worry makes difficult.

Steps:

1. Begin on hands and knees, wrists under shoulders, knees under hips.
2. Extend your right arm forward while your left leg reaches back.
3. Hold for 3-5 breaths, focusing on maintaining balance and core engagement.
4. Return slowly to the starting position.
5. Repeat with left arm forward and right leg back.
6. Complete 5-10 repetitions on each side, moving with control and awareness.

Sphinx Pose

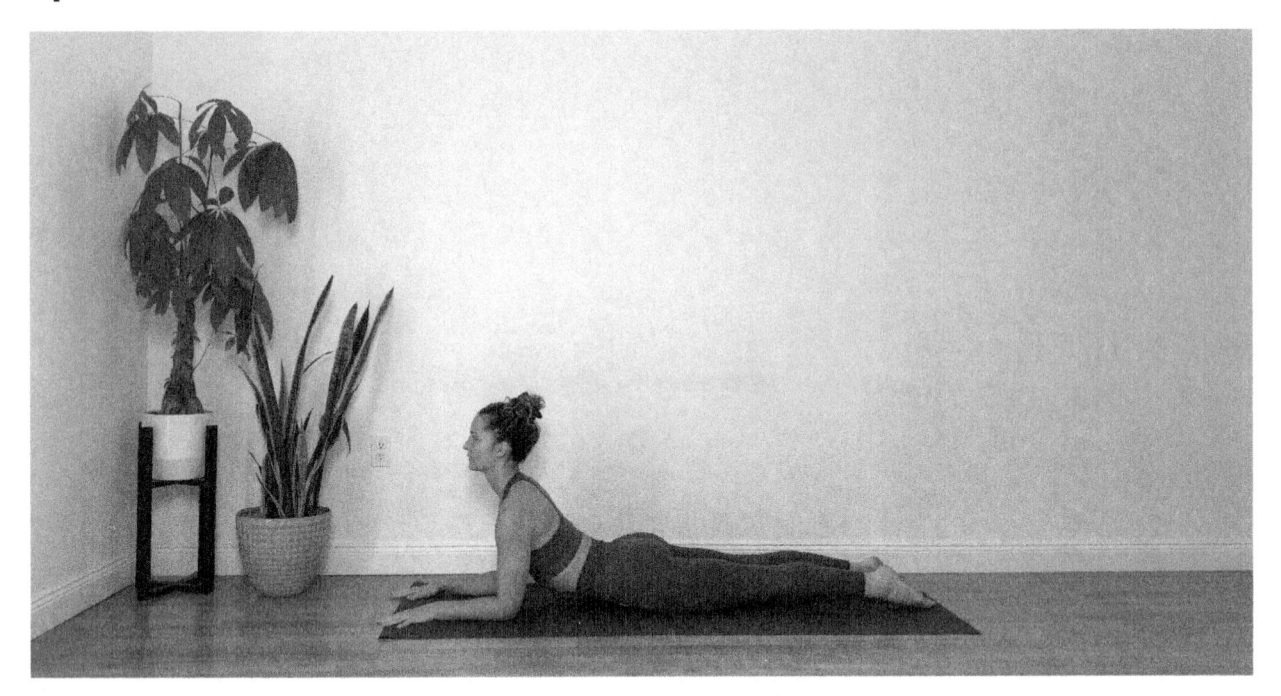

This gentle backbend creates space in areas where anxiety causes constriction. By opening the chest and supporting the spine, you physically counteract the collapsed posture that both reflects and reinforces stress.

Steps:

1. Lie on your stomach with legs extended.
2. Place your elbows under your shoulders, forearms on the floor.
3. Lift your upper body while keeping your hips and legs grounded.
4. Draw your shoulder blades down your back as your chest opens forward.
5. Keep your gaze forward or slightly downward to maintain proper neck alignment.
6. Hold for 5-10 deep breaths, focusing on chest expansion with each inhale.
7. Gradually lower your upper body back to the floor to release.
8. Rest briefly before repeating 2-3 times if comfortable.

Side-Lying Leg Lifts

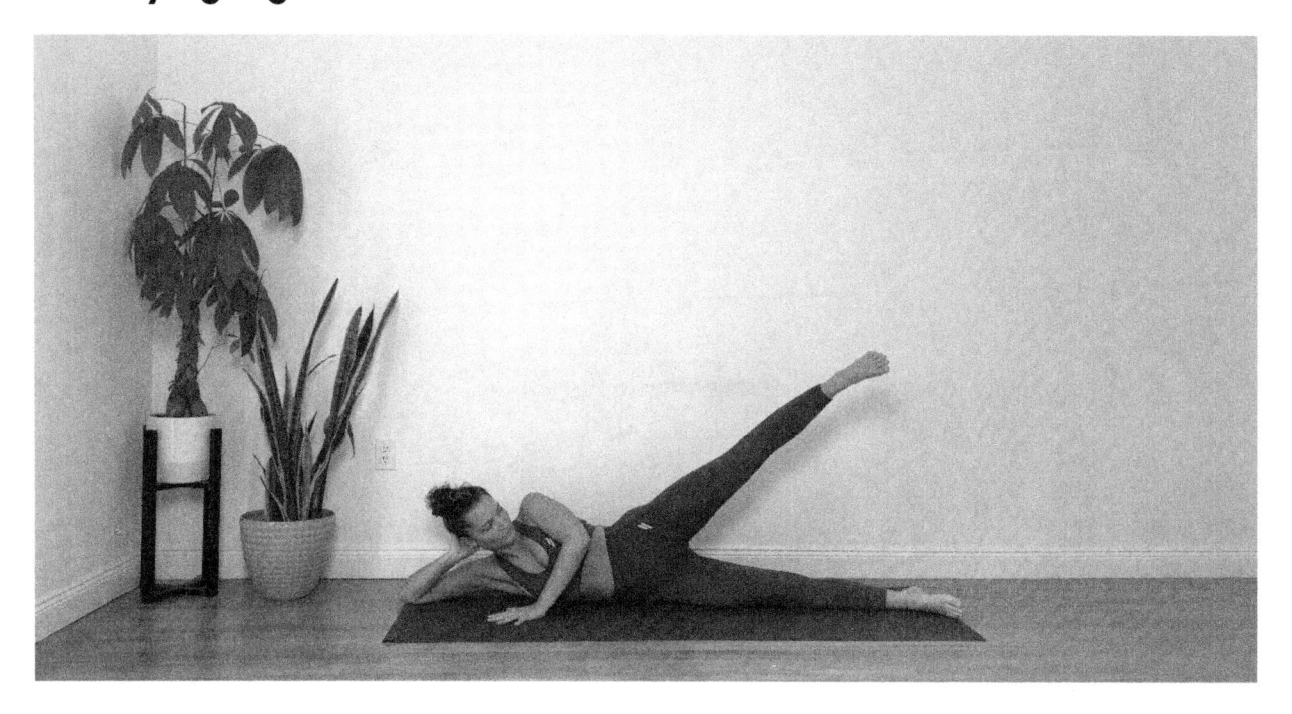

These leg lifts engage the outer hip muscles that modern living often leaves dormant. This movement isn't just for strength—it's a way to reestablish a connection with your foundation that daily stress can disrupt.

1. Position yourself on your right side, legs aligned and slightly bent at the knees.
2. Support your head with your right hand or rest it comfortably on your arm.
3. Stabilize your torso by placing your left palm on the floor ahead of you.
4. Maintaining stacked hips, deliberately raise your left leg to about 45 degrees.
5. Pause briefly at the peak, then lower with control.
6. Complete 10-15 mindful repetitions.
7. Transition to your left side and repeat the sequence with your right leg.
8. Use each movement as an anchor for your attention, noticing the sensation rather than letting thoughts wander.

Somatic Shoulder Shrugs

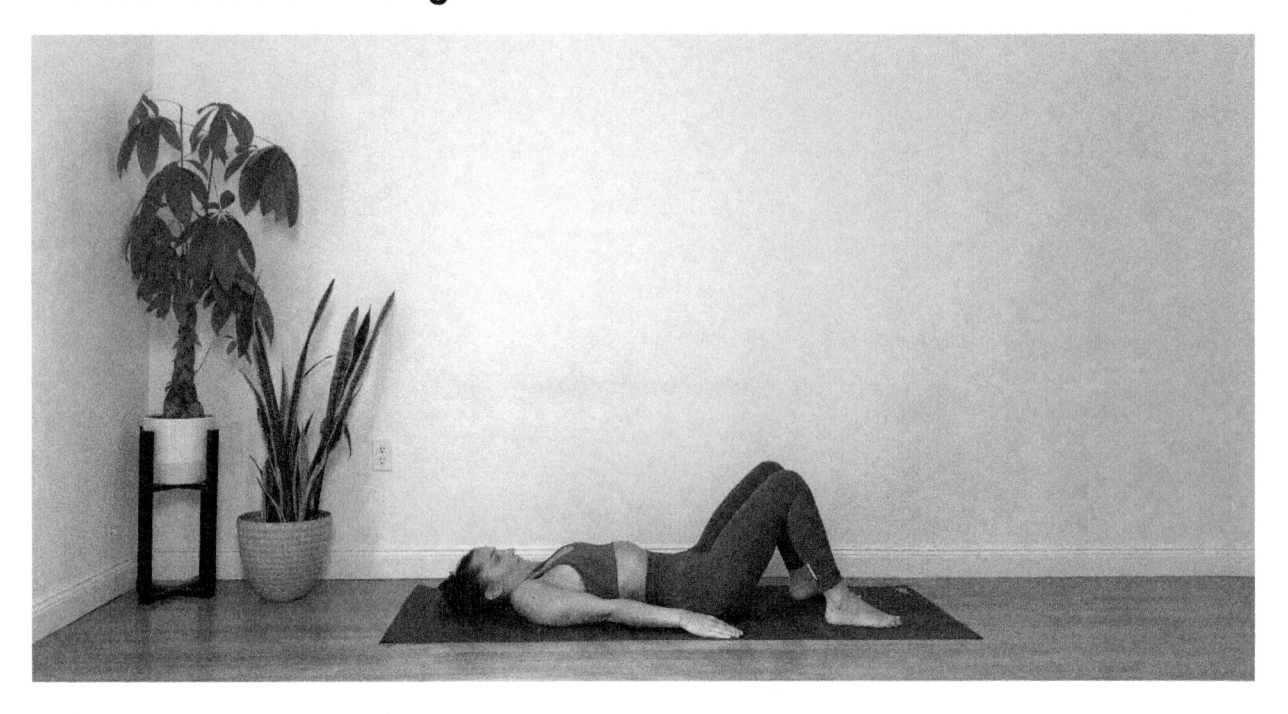

Your shoulders collect the tension of decisions unmade and responsibilities carried. This exercise helps release what you've been holding, creating space where restriction has become normal.

1. Lie down on your back, knees bent with feet grounded on the floor.
2. Allow your arms to settle beside you, palms connecting with the surface.
3. As you draw breath in, gradually lift your shoulders toward your ears.
4. With your exhale, release them downward, allowing them to surrender to gravity.
5. Bring full attention to the contrast between engagement and release.
6. Continue this mindful cycle for 10-15 breaths, staying connected to your body's rhythm.
7. After completing the final movement, let your shoulders fully release and notice the difference.

Breathing Techniques for Anxiety Management

Your breath—simple, steady, and underappreciated—holds a secret power. We do it thousands of times a day, yet when we take control, it's like flipping a switch on anxiety. It's your anchor, your lifeline, always there, always ready to ground you when the world gets loud.

When anxiety barges in, your breath can turn into a shallow, panicked mess, feeding that constant loop of tension. But guess what? You can take control. Deep, slow breaths send a clear message to your nervous system: "We're good. No need to go into survival mode." You are essentially instructing your body to stop its fight-or-flight response. It functions similarly to a reset button for your entire system.

What's the best part? It's simple. No fancy settings, no special devices. Your breath is there whether you're stuck in a subway vehicle, have a deadline to meet, or are staring at the ceiling at three in the morning. A silent hero in your battle against anxiety, always ready to help you find that calm space amidst the storm.

This section is your toolkit. A mix of practical breathing techniques to tap into your superpower, the one you've been carrying around this whole time. You've got this. Let's breathe our way to peace.

Box Breathing (Square Breathing)

This structured breathing pattern helps reset a nervous system that's forgotten how to rest. The even counts create balance in a system that may have been running on emergency mode for too long.

1. Find a comfortable seated position that supports your spine.
2. Empty your lungs completely with a deliberate exhale.
3. Draw breath in through your nose for a steady count of 4.
4. Retain this breath for an equal count of 4.
5. Release the breath through your mouth for 4 counts.
6. Hold empty for a count of 4 before beginning again.
7. Continue this rhythmic pattern for 4-5 minutes, or until you notice a shift toward calm.

SOMATIC EXERCISES FOR NERVOUS SYSTEM REGULATION

4-7-8 Breathing

Dr. Weil's technique works directly with your nervous system's natural design, helping shift from the stress response that modern life keeps activated to the rest response your body craves.

1. Sit with your spine supported and aligned.
2. Position your tongue just behind your upper front teeth.
3. Release all breath through your mouth with an audible whoosh.
4. Draw breath in quietly through your nose for a count of 4.
5. Hold this breath, maintaining awareness for a count of 7.
6. Exhale completely through your mouth with another audible whoosh for a count of 8.
7. Complete 4 full cycles of this pattern.

Alternate Nostril Breathing (Nadi Shodhana)

This yogic technique helps balance your system by alternating breath between nostrils. It serves as a reset for the mind-body connection when stress has created an imbalance.

1. Sit comfortably with your spine naturally aligned.
2. Close your right nostril using your right thumb.
3. Inhale fully through your open left nostril.
4. At inhalation's peak, close the left nostril with your ring finger, release the right, and exhale through the right pathway.
5. Inhale through this same right nostril.
6. At full inhalation, close the right side and exhale through the left.
7. This completes one full cycle. Continue for 5-10 cycles.

Deep Belly Breathing (Diaphragmatic Breathing)

Most of us have forgotten how to breathe fully, adopting shallow chest breathing that signals stress to our bodies. This practice reawakens the natural, deep breathing pattern that signals safety to your nervous system.

1. Lie back with knees bent, feet planted on the floor.
2. Place one hand on your chest and the other just below your ribcage.

CHAPTER 4: MANAGING ANXIETY WITH SOMATIC EXERCISE

3. Inhale slowly through your nose, allowing your belly to rise against your lower hand while your chest hand remains relatively still.
4. Engage your abdominal muscles as you exhale through pursed lips, feeling your stomach draw inward. Keep your chest and hand stable.
5. Continue this conscious breathing pattern for 5-10 minutes.

Here's the deal: practice is the magic ingredient in any exercise. It's gonna feel weird at first, like trying to get used to a new pair of shoes. But stick with it, and soon enough, these techniques will flow like second nature. The key? Start when you're calm—because that's when you can really own these tools. When anxiety hits, you'll be able to access them like a ninja, and trust me, that's what you want.

And don't forget to breathe at a pace that feels like it fits, okay? No need to force it—this isn't a race. If it feels uncomfortable, back off a bit. Your body knows the way; let it guide you.

Chapter 5: Stress Relief Through Somatic Exercise

Move your body to free your mind; in physical release lies mental peace.

Here's a fun fact: At rest, our bodies carry enough energy to power a small city. Now, I'm no scientist (just a writer with a flair for thinking), but the evidence here is clear: we're all like tiny walking power plants, buzzing with energy. And you know what? I really believe that we are all responsible for keeping the lights on at night.

But that energy sometimes? It becomes a bit... erratic. Instead of illuminating the planet, we are short-circuiting our own systems as we transform into walking, talking electrical bundles. Ever had one of those days where even the smallest task feels like climbing Everest? Where your brain is buzzing louder than a swarm of angry bees? That's your personal power plant going haywire.

I'm not saying we need to shut down our power stations. What we need is to find a way to channel that energy and smooth out the spikes and dips. You don't need more stress; you need balance. You listen to your body, find where the energy is stuck, and guide it back into a steady flow. In this chapter, we'll talk about how mindful movements can transform that chaotic lightning storm into a steady, warm glow.

External and Internal Stressors

We've got two radars working 24/7: one scanning the world around us, the other keeping tabs on what's going on inside our heads. Let's break down what each one picks up:

External Stressors

These come from outside us—stuff we can't always control but that still hits like a ton of bricks. These are the things in your environment that push your stress buttons.

Examples:

- Work pressure (deadlines, tough bosses, heavy workloads)
- Financial pressure (debt, surprise expenses, job loss)

- Relationship pressure (fights with partners, family, friends)
- Major life changes (moving, getting hitched, having a baby)
- Environmental noise (traffic, crowded spaces, bad weather)
- The state of the world (political mess, disasters, pandemics)
- Time crunches (too many things to do, not enough time)
- Traffic (ugh, just... traffic)
- Social pressures (keeping up with everyone)
- Academic stressors (exams, applications, stress)

These external stressors? The ones we vent about with friends or post on social media. They are palpable, observable, and extremely communicable. "That right there?" we can remark, pointing to them. "I'm stressed out because of that."

Internal Stressors

Let's go on to the more covert ones, the internal pressures. Instead of coming from the outside, these come from within. And trust me, they're often far more challenging to deal with.

Examples:

- Negative self-talk (yes, that constant inner critic)
- Perfectionism, or striving for an unachievable ideal
- Being pessimistic (believing that everything is half-empty)
- Fear (of everything, really, including failure and success)
- Shame or guilt over the past (like having extra luggage)
- Low self-esteem (feeling inadequate)
- Future uncertainty (a sense of being lost)
- Lack of control, or the perception that life is controlling you rather than the other way around
- Unresolved feelings or trauma from the past (like a replaying broken record)
- The practice of delaying everything is known as procrastination.

These internal stressors are sneaky because they often stay hidden, buried in your mind. They're the things that keep you up at night, worried about things that haven't even happened yet or reliving previous errors. However, you'll be more capable of handling pressures once you can recognize both internal and external ones. You can control everything, whether that means altering your environment, changing the way you think, or employing somatic exercises to relieve the tension that has been stored in your body.

Techniques for Identifying Your Personal Stressors

Let's talk about the art of catching stress in its natural habitat. Think of it like a scavenger hunt, where you're piecing together clues, spotting patterns, and catching yourself red-handed mid-stress. It takes some work, yeah, but it's like sharpening a tool that gets more effective the more you use it. Here's how you can do it:

The Body Scan Method

Your body's the unsung hero here—it's often clued in before your mind even knows what's going on. Here's how to tap into that wisdom:

- Carve out a few minutes daily to mentally scan yourself, head to toe.
- Pay attention to any tight spots, discomfort, or random sensations.
- Ask yourself: What was going on in my head when I felt this tension?

This method links physical stress signs to their triggers, so you'll start seeing stress coming from miles away.

The Stress Journal

Keeping a stress journal is like shining a spotlight on your stress patterns. Here's the drill:

- Every day, jot down any stressful moments and how you reacted.
- Be specific—time, place, people involved, and how your body and mind were feeling.
- After a week or two, go back and review. Look for recurring themes, like certain places or people always being stress triggers.
- You'll be surprised at how these small notes can reveal the big picture. It's like you're reading your stress blueprint.

The "What If" Game

Sometimes, stress isn't really about the present but the anxiety about the future. Want to dissect that? Try this:

- When you're feeling anxious, ask yourself, What am I afraid might happen?
- Then follow it up with, What if that happened? Keep going with this, layering the "What ifs" until you uncover what you're worried about.

This will help you separate the realistic fears from the ones that are a product of your imagination. Most of your worries might just be unlikely scenarios!

The Energy Audit

It's not just about what's draining you—it's about where that drain is coming from. Here's the approach:

- Throughout the day, pay attention to activities or interactions that make you feel drained or tense.
- Also, make a note of the moments that leave you feeling energized or relaxed.
- At the end of the day, look at the rundown. The energy-draining activities? Yeah, they're probably your stressors.

Think of this as a stress energy map that leads you to the source of the chaos.

The Mindful Pause

Catching stress in real-time? That's the power move. Here's how:

- Several times a day, especially when switching between tasks, take a deliberate pause.
- During that moment, check in with your thoughts, emotions, and body sensations.
- If you're feeling stressed, ask yourself: What's contributing to this feeling right now?

This practice can help you stop stress before it snowballs into full-blown chaos.

The Trusted Friend Perspective

Sometimes, we're too deep in our own lives to see the bigger picture. So, get someone else's eyes on it:

CHAPTER 5: STRESS RELIEF THROUGH SOMATIC EXERCISE

- Tell a trusted friend about your day or week.
- Ask them if they see any recurring stress patterns in your routine.

Their outside perspective can shine a light on stressors you've been too close to recognize.

The Values Checklist

Stress often creeps in when our actions are out of sync with what matters to us. Here's how to check:
- Make a list of your core values (family, career, creativity, health, etc.).
- Look at your daily activities and see how well they align with these values.
- Notice any areas where your actions don't match up. Those misalignments? Major stress red flags.

If what you're doing doesn't reflect what you truly value, that's where the stress is hiding.

Somatic Exercises for Relaxation

Your body holds your emotional state like a tight grip, but you can loosen it up with mindful movement. Somatic exercises are designed to release that tension, boost your body awareness, and help you hit that sweet spot of calm.

These exercises are gentle, accessible, and perfect for all levels. They're your ticket to taking control of both your body and mind, leaving you feeling balanced, grounded, and ready to tackle whatever comes your way.

SOMATIC EXERCISES FOR NERVOUS SYSTEM REGULATION

Standing Wall Roll Down

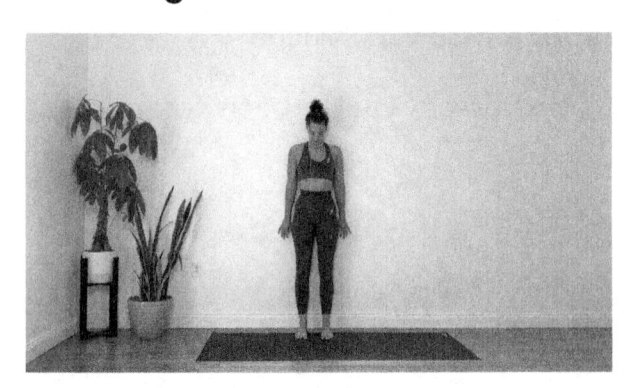

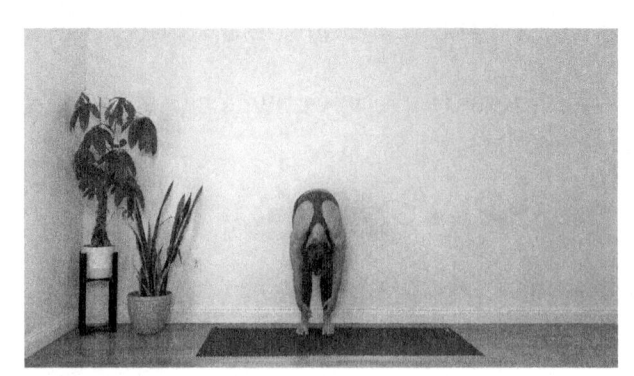

This exercise helps free your spine from the rigidity that stress creates throughout the day. By deliberately moving through each vertebra, you reconnect with parts of your back that have become locked in patterns of tension and disconnect.

Position yourself with your back against a wall, feet hip-width apart and about 6 inches from the wall.

1. Begin with your entire back, shoulders, and head in contact with the wall.
2. Inhale deeply. As you exhale, begin by tucking your chin and then gradually peel your spine away from the wall, one vertebra at a time.
3. Continue this controlled unraveling until your upper body hangs toward the floor, or as far as feels appropriate for your body.
4. Pause briefly, allowing your back muscles to experience the release of habitual holding.
5. With your next inhale, begin the deliberate process of rolling back up, each vertebra finding its place against the wall until you're fully upright.
6. Once vertical again, take a full breath and notice the renewed length in your spine.
7. Repeat this conscious movement 5-10 times, synchronizing with your breath's natural rhythm.

Supine Arm Circles

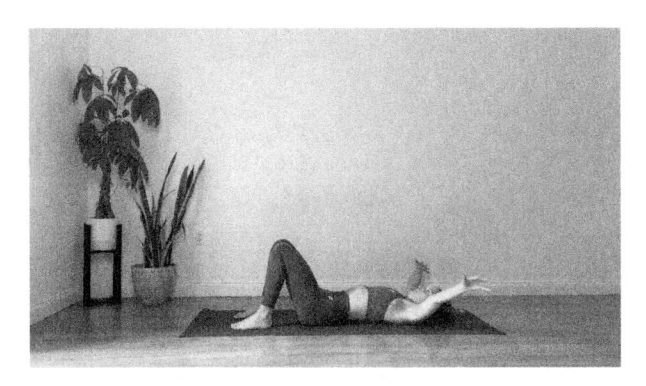

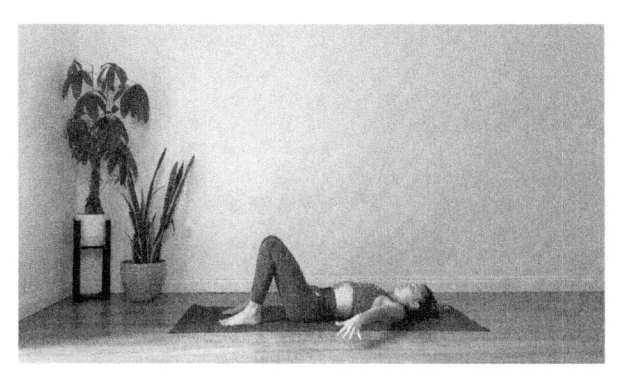

The shoulders often carry the tension of responsibilities and worries that go unaddressed. These gentle circles help release what's been stored in your upper body, creating freedom where restriction has become the norm.

1. Lie back with knees bent, feet grounded on the floor.
2. Extend your arms outward to form a T-shape with your torso.
3. Begin making small, deliberate circles with your arms while maintaining contact with the floor.
4. Gradually increase the circle size, staying within a comfortable range for your shoulders.
5. After completing 5-10 circles in one direction, reverse the pattern.
6. Coordinate with your breath—inhale as your arms move upward and exhale as they travel down.
7. Continue this rhythmic movement for 1-2 minutes or as long as feels beneficial.

Somatic Sunbird Pose

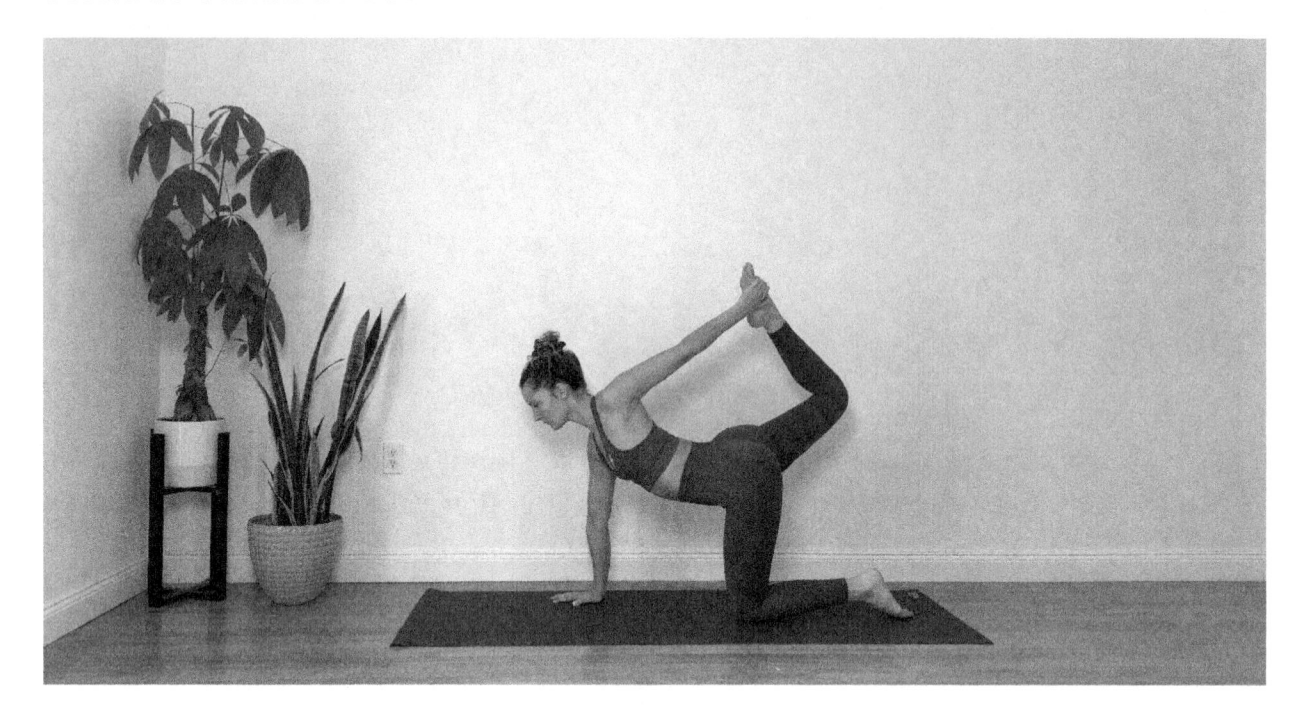

This balanced extension helps bring awareness to your core center while creating stability in a world that often feels ungrounded. The coordination required brings attention fully to the present moment, away from anxious thoughts.

1. Begin in tabletop position, wrists aligned under shoulders and knees under hips.
2. With deliberate control, extend your right arm forward as your left leg reaches backward.
3. Maintain your center by keeping your spine neutral, avoiding arching or twisting.
4. Hold this balanced position for 3-5 complete breaths, focusing on the sensation of stability.
5. Return mindfully to your starting position.
6. Mirror this movement with your left arm and right leg extended.
7. Alternate sides for 5-10 repetitions each, moving with awareness rather than speed.

Somatic Hip Rolls

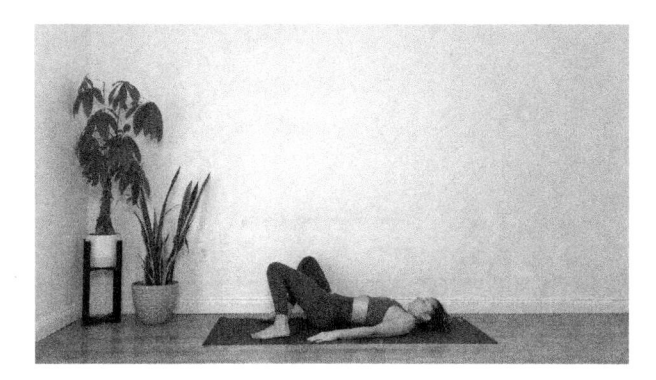

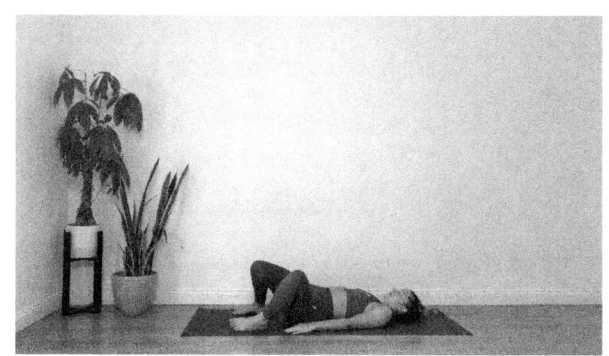

The hips and lower back become repositories for unprocessed stress. These gentle rolls help release tension that many of us store without realizing, reconnecting us with our foundation.

1. Lie down on your back, knees bent with feet planted hip-width apart.
2. Position arms slightly outward, palms down for support.
3. Gently engage your core to create contact between your lower back and the floor.
4. Begin a slow, controlled roll of your hips rightward, allowing your knees to lower toward the floor as feels comfortable.
5. Pause momentarily, then deliberately return to center.
6. Continue this movement to the left side.
7. Alternate sides for 5-10 repetitions in each direction.
8. Pay attention to sensations in your hips and lower back, noticing areas of holding or release.

Lying Hip Release

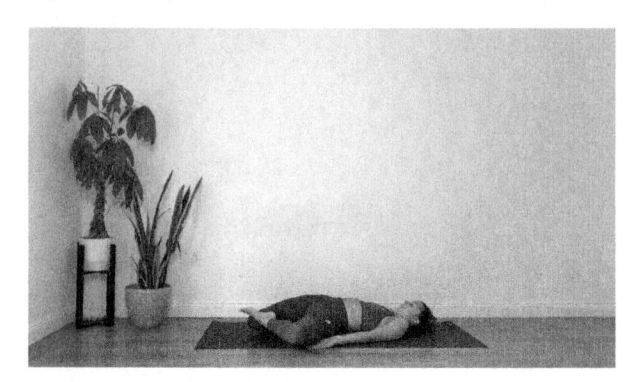

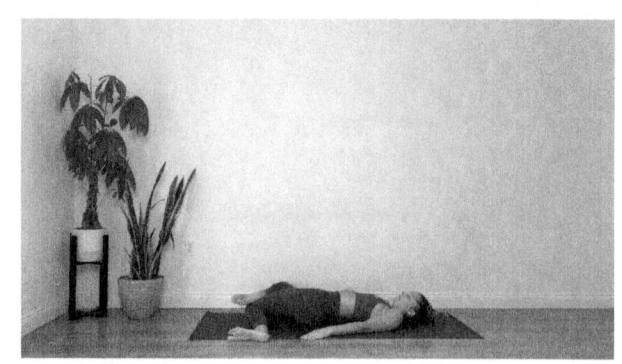

Your hips hold the tension of modern life—from long periods of sitting to stress responses that tighten these crucial joints. This gentle opening creates space where compression has become normal.

1. Lie back with knees bent, feet grounded at hip-width.
2. Allow your arms to rest alongside you, palms connecting with the floor.
3. With gentleness, let your knees fall naturally to one side while keeping your feet on the floor.
4. Remain here for 5-10 full breaths, noticing the opening across your hip and lower back.
5. With awareness, return to center before repeating on the opposite side.
6. Continue this alternating pattern for 3-5 repetitions on each side.

CHAPTER 5: STRESS RELIEF THROUGH SOMATIC EXERCISE

Somatic Wave

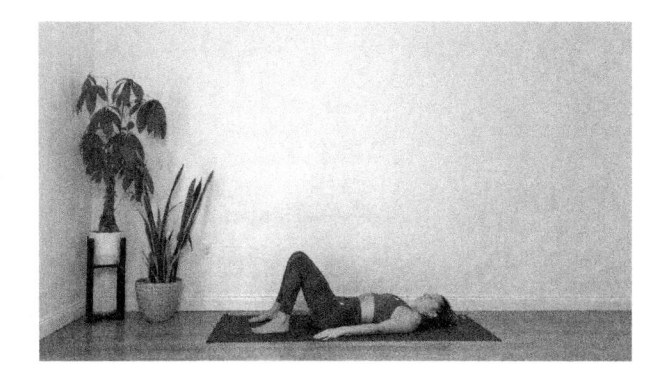

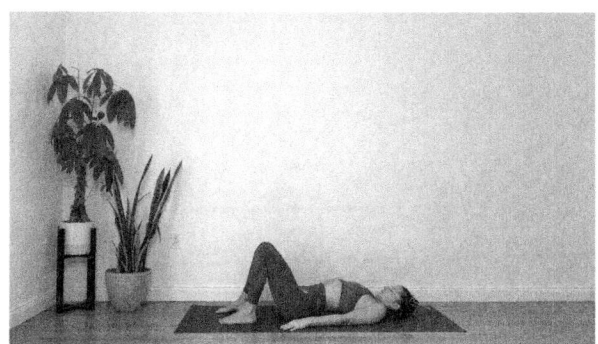

This fluid motion reintroduces your spine to movement it may have forgotten. By creating a wave through your central column, you reawaken communication between segments that have become isolated by tension.

1. Lie down on your back with your knees bent and feet planted on the floor.
2. Initiate movement by tucking your tailbone and gradually rolling your spine upward off the floor, one vertebra at a time.
3. Continue this controlled articulation until you reach your shoulder blades.
4. Pause briefly at the peak, then begin the mindful descent, each vertebra reconnecting with the floor.
5. Pay close attention to the sensation of each segment making contact with the surface beneath you.
6. Repeat this flowing movement 5-10 times, moving with deliberate awareness.

Standing Pelvic Tilts

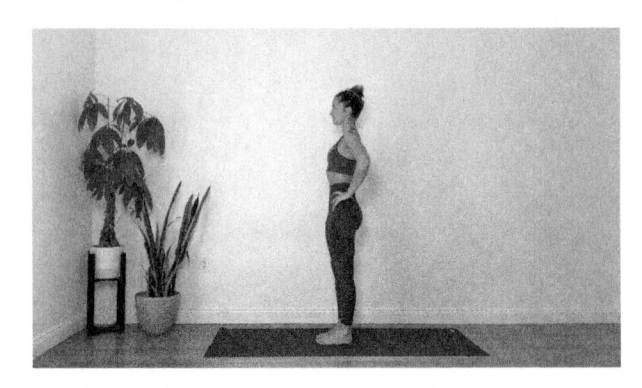

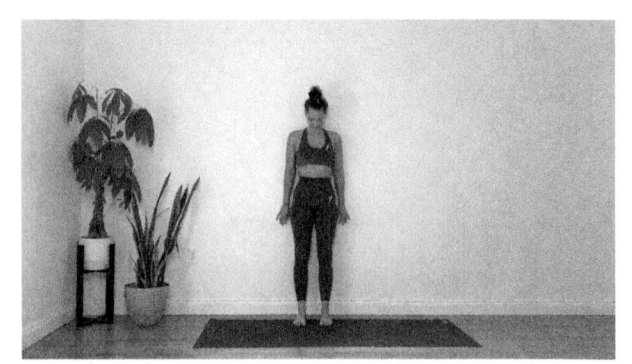

This exercise invites you to reclaim the natural movement of your pelvis, an area where we often hold the tension of our busy days. By consciously directing this gentle rocking motion, you're releasing patterns of holding that can contribute to lower back discomfort and disconnection from your center.

1. Stand with your feet hip-width apart, knees slightly softened to release unnecessary tension.
2. Rest your hands on your hips, allowing your fingertips to become sensors of the subtle movement to come.
3. As you exhale, slowly tilt your pelvis forward, feeling how this action gently arches your lower back.
4. With your next breath, tilt your pelvis backward, noticing how this movement creates a flattening sensation in your lower spine.
5. Continue this mindful rocking motion, paying attention to how the movement ripples through your entire body.
6. Repeat for 10-15 cycles, synchronizing each tilt with the natural rhythm of your breath.

Dynamic Warrior I

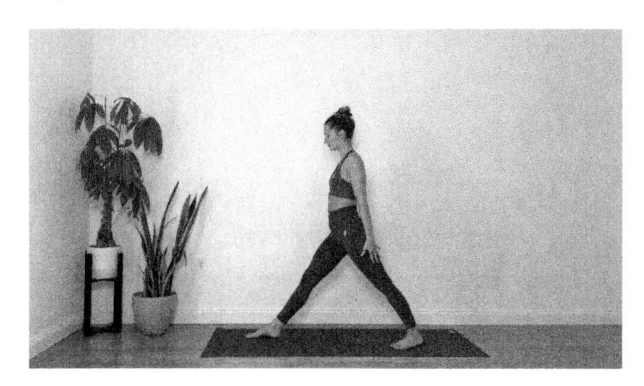

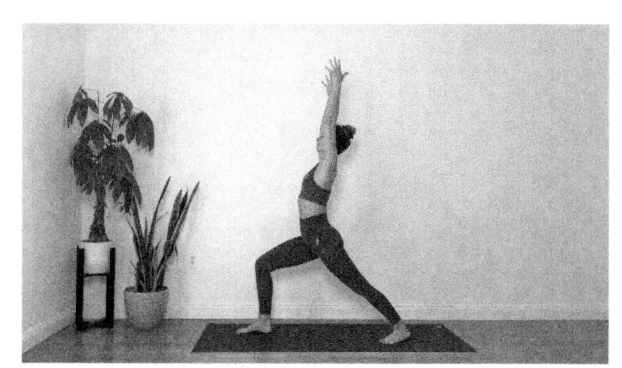

The warrior stance embodies both strength and surrender – qualities we need to navigate daily life. This flowing variation helps release the armor we build around our hips and chest, areas where we store unprocessed emotions and experiences.

Begin in a centered standing position, feeling your connection to the ground beneath you.

1. Step your left foot back approximately 3-4 feet, allowing it to find a comfortable 45-degree angle.

2. Bend into your right knee, ensuring it stacks directly above your ankle to protect your joint.

3. As you draw breath in, let your arms rise overhead, allowing a gentle expansion through your chest and a slight arching in your back.

4. With your exhale, release your arms downward as you straighten your front leg, creating a wave-like motion through your entire body.

5. Continue this rhythmic flowing movement, letting each breath guide the timing of your expansion and release.

6. Complete 5-10 full cycles before mindfully transitioning to the opposite side.

Somatic Warrior II

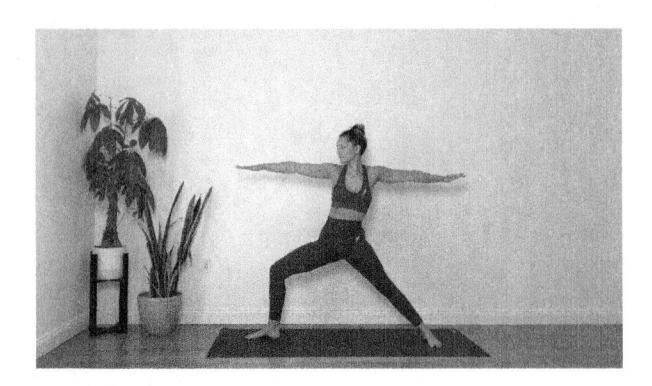

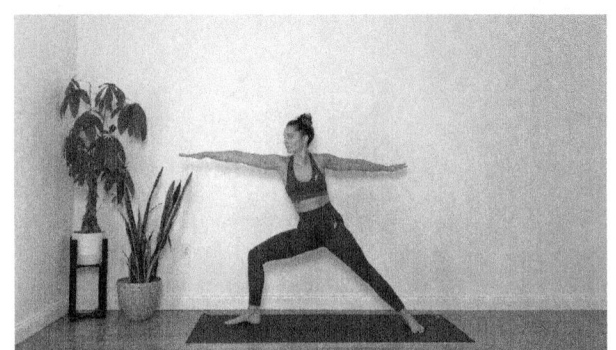

This variation invites you to explore the subtle sensations within a powerful stance. By introducing gentle movement, you're breaking through habitual holding patterns and awakening new awareness in areas that have become rigid or numb.

1. Create a wide foundation by stepping your feet apart, turning your right foot outward 90 degrees while your left foot rotates slightly inward.

2. Bend into your right knee, creating a strong base while maintaining alignment above your ankle.

3. Extend your arms outward at shoulder height, feeling the opposing energies moving through your fingertips.

4. Begin a gentle swaying motion with your upper body, noticing how this shifts the weight distribution through your legs and feet.

5. Bring your attention to the changing sensations in your legs, hips, and shoulders as you move, noticing areas of holding or freedom.

6. Maintain this mindful exploration for 30-60 seconds before honoring the other side of your body with the same attention.

Gentle Standing Twists

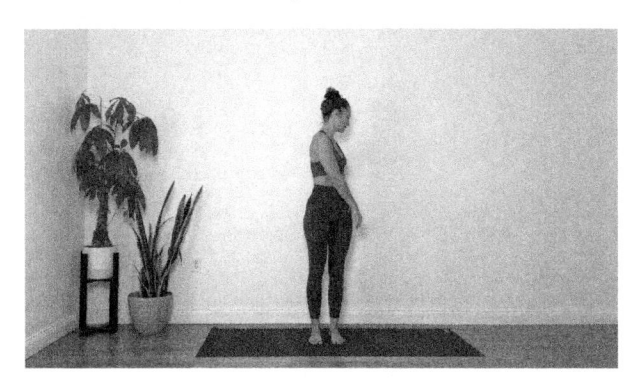

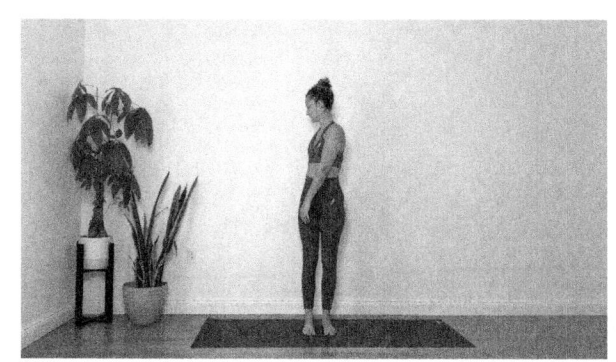

The spine houses not only our nervous system but also holds the residue of unexpressed emotions and stress. These twists help unwind the accumulated tension while promoting the healthy mobility that allows energy to flow more freely throughout your body.

1. Stand with your feet hip-width apart, knees slightly softened to remove unnecessary tension.
2. Allow your arms to hang naturally at your sides, surrendering to gravity.
3. Initiate a gentle twist from your center to the right, permitting your arms to follow this rotation with their natural momentum.
4. Then invite your body to unwind and rotate toward the left, again allowing your arms to respond to this movement without forcing.
5. Maintain a slow, deliberate pace, focusing on the sensation of each vertebra participating in this releasing motion.
6. Continue for 10-15 cycles, allowing your breath to naturally complement this unwinding movement.

SOMATIC EXERCISES FOR NERVOUS SYSTEM REGULATION

Dynamic Tree Pose

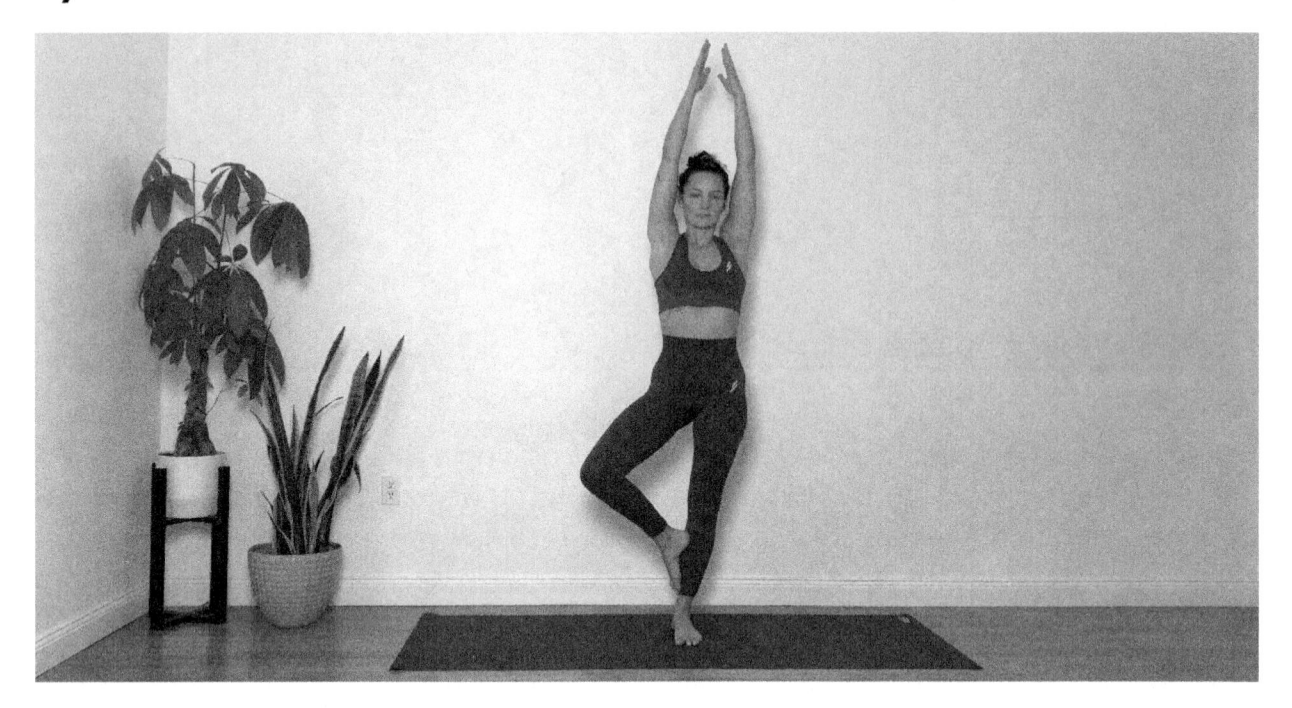

This flowing variation of the Tree Pose helps us practice finding center amidst movement, just as we must in our daily lives. The rhythmic rising and lowering mirrors the natural cycles of growth and rest that govern all living things.

1. Ground through your left leg, bringing awareness to the three points of contact your foot makes with the earth.

2. Gently place your right foot against your left inner thigh or calf, honoring your body's current flexibility (avoiding pressure on the knee).

3. As you draw breath in, let your arms rise skyward, embodying the upward growth of a tree reaching toward light.

4. With your exhale, mindfully lower both your arms and right foot, returning to your rooted standing position.

5. Repeat this flowing sequence 5-10 times, focusing on the dialogue between stability in your standing leg and the freedom of movement above.

6. Honor both sides of your body by repeating this practice with the opposite foot.

Somatic Forward Fold

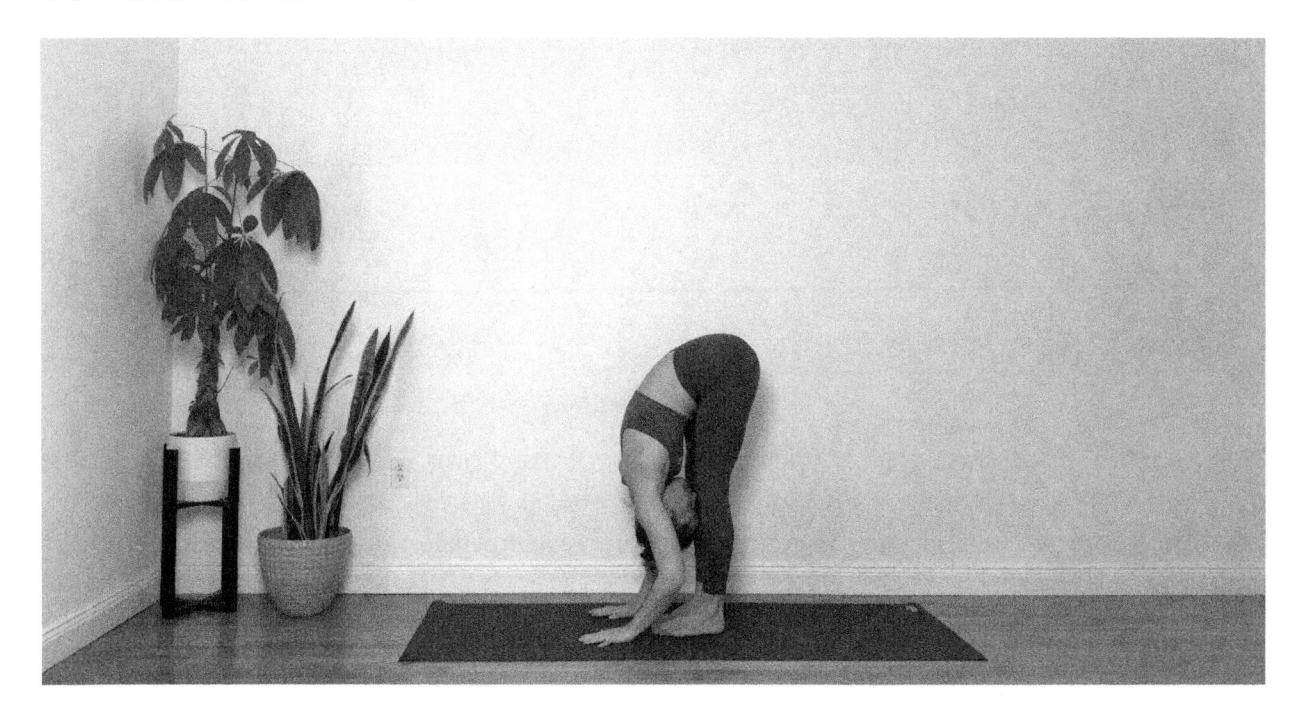

This movement invites surrender—a conscious release of the tension we carry in our back body and the mental burdens we hold. By moving between extension and folding, you're practicing the balance of effort and ease that characterizes a healthy relationship with your body.

1. Stand with your feet hip-width apart, knees slightly softened to protect your lower back.
2. Inhale deeply as you extend your arms overhead, creating length through your entire spine.
3. As you release your breath, begin folding forward from your hip creases, allowing your upper body to surrender to gravity.
4. Let your head and arms hang heavy, creating space for your back muscles to release their habitual patterns of holding.
5. With your next inhale, initiate a mindful rolling-up motion, stacking each vertebra thoughtfully until you've returned to standing.
6. Repeat this flowing movement 5-7 times, moving with the natural rhythm of your breath and honoring your body's wisdom.

Chair Pose with Arm Waves

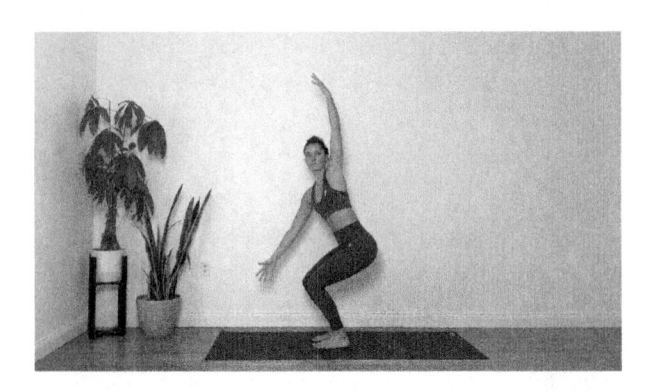

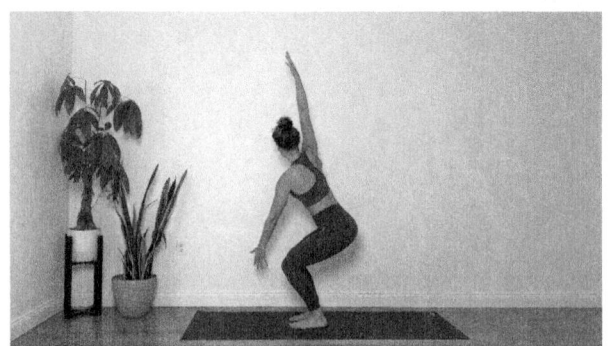

This practice combines the grounding stability of the Chair Pose with the fluid release of wave-like arm movements. This contrast helps release the tension we hold in our shoulders while building awareness of our capacity to be both strong and fluid simultaneously.

1. Stand with your feet rooted hip-width apart, feeling the even distribution of weight through your feet.

2. Bend your knees and lower your hips backward as if being invited to sit, creating engagement through your lower body.

3. Extend your arms upward, creating length through the sides of your waist.

4. While maintaining the stability in your lower body, begin a flowing, alternating motion with your arms – as one rises, the other descends.

5. Allow this wavelike movement to release tension in your shoulders and chest, areas where we often store stress and unexpressed emotions.

6. Continue this rhythmic practice for 30-60 seconds, noticing the interplay between the stability of your legs and the freedom in your upper body.

Somatic Side Stretch

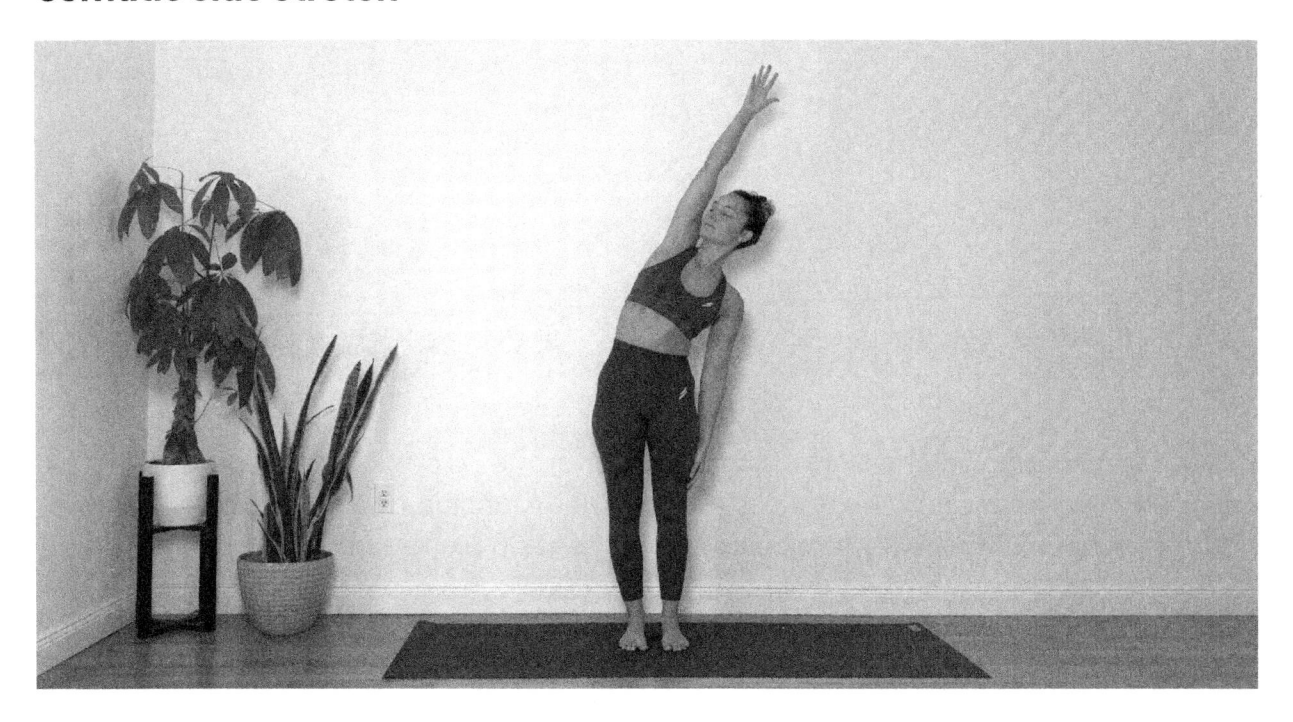

The sides of our bodies often become compressed through daily activities and emotional holding. This mindful stretch creates space between each rib, inviting fuller breath and releasing constriction in areas that rarely receive our conscious attention.

1. Stand with your feet planted hip-width apart, establishing a stable foundation.

2. Extend your right arm skyward, allowing your left arm to rest naturally at your side.

3. Initiate a gentle lateral curve to the left, creating length along the entire right side of your body from hip to fingertips.

4. Remain here for 2-3 full breath cycles, noticing how the ribcage expands and contracts with each breath.

5. Mindfully return to center before repeating this expansive movement on the opposite side.

6. Continue alternating between sides for 5-7 repetitions, noticing if one side feels different from the other – a valuable insight into your body's unique patterns.

Dynamic Downward Dog

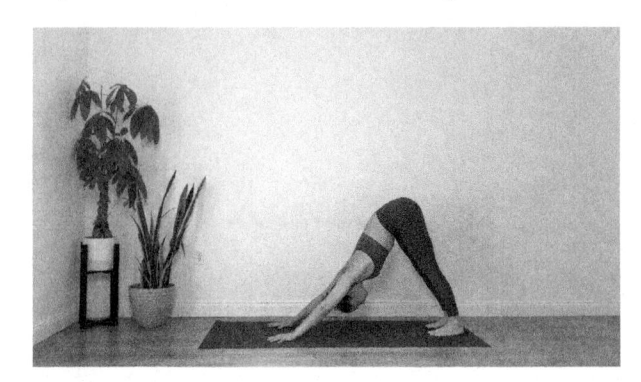

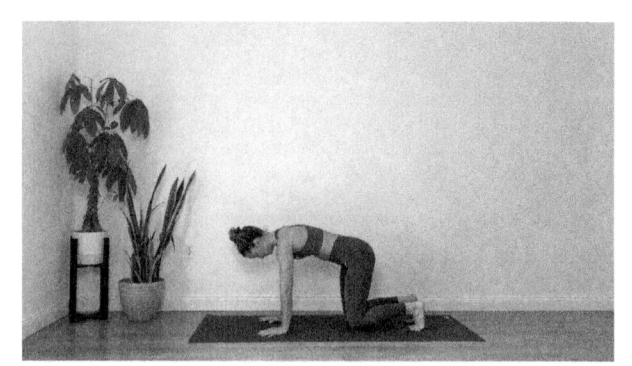

This flowing variation of the Downward Dog encourages a conversation between effort and surrender, mimicking the natural rhythms of expansion and contraction that exist in all living things. The movement helps release tension along the entire posterior chain of the body.

1. Begin in a tabletop position, with your awareness distributed evenly through your hands and knees.

2. As you exhale, lift your hips skyward while straightening your arms and legs, creating the inverted V-shape of Downward Dog.

3. Pause for a full breath cycle, feeling the lengthening through your spine and the opening across the backs of your legs.

4. With your next inhale, mindfully release back to the tabletop position, surrendering any unnecessary holding.

5. Continue flowing between these positions for 5-7 cycles, letting each movement be guided by the natural rhythm of your breath.

6. Notice the sensations of alternating between effort and ease, a microcosm of how we might move through our daily lives with more awareness.

Somatic Crescent Lunge

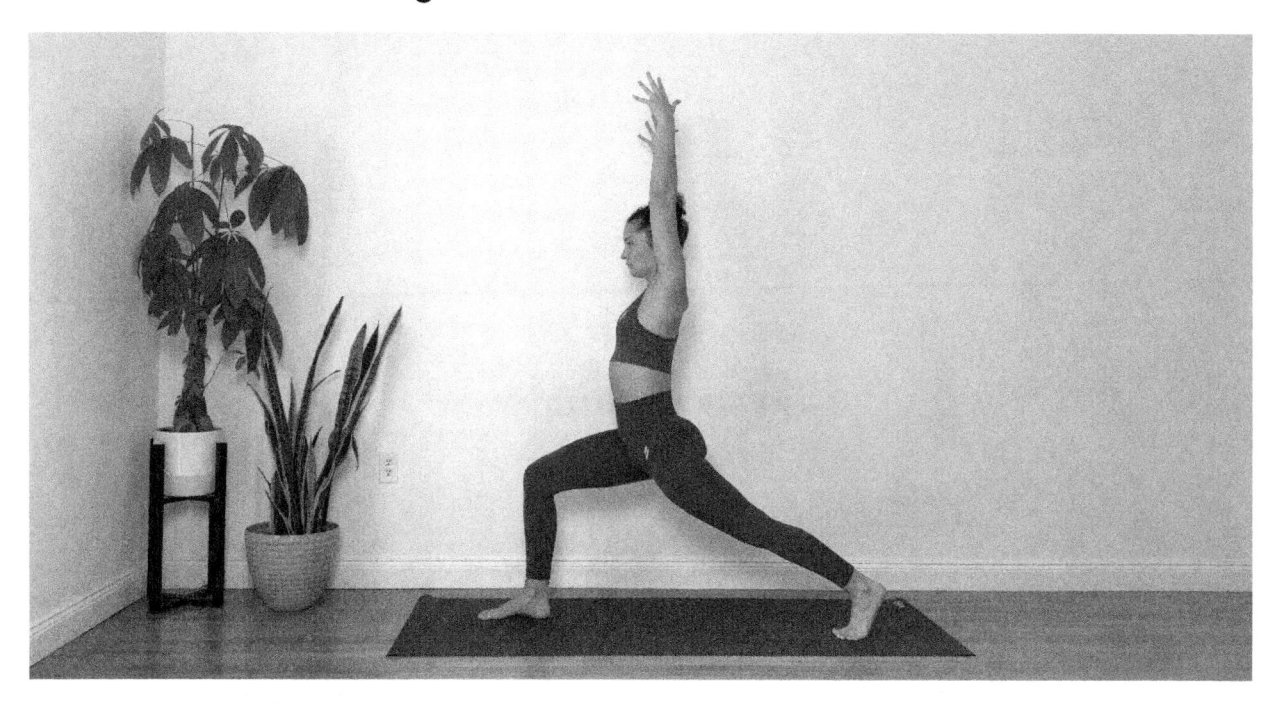

This variation explores the subtle movements available within a strong foundation. The hip flexors often store tension related to our stress response, and this mindful practice helps release this deeply held pattern while encouraging new awareness in this vital area.

1. From a centered standing position, step your right foot back, creating length between your feet.
2. Bend into your left knee, ensuring it stacks above your ankle as you establish this lunging position.
3. Extend your arms upward, creating length through your torso and openness across your chest.
4. Begin a gentle swaying motion from side to side, noticing how this subtle movement creates changing sensations throughout your hips and legs.
5. After exploring these lateral movements, introduce small, pulsing movements up and down, moving just an inch or two to release deeper layers of tension.
6. Continue this exploratory practice for 30-60 seconds before mindfully transitioning to nurture the opposite side.

Reclined Butterfly Pose

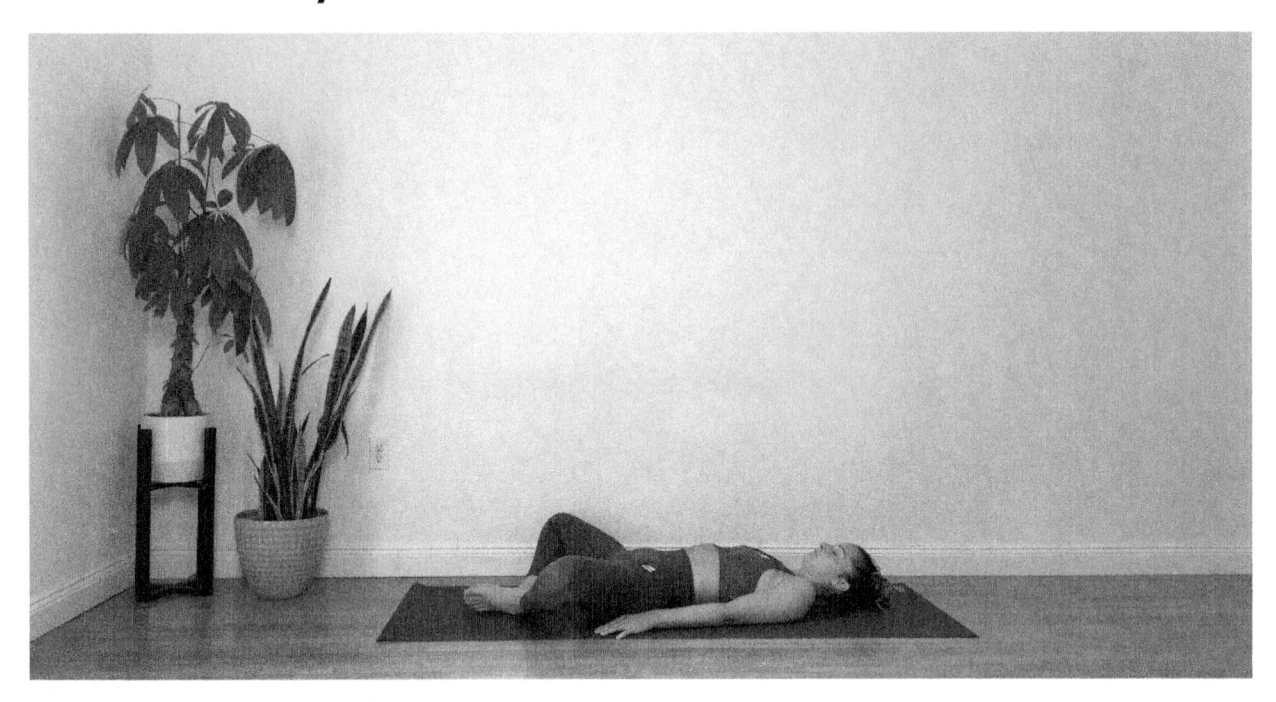

This restorative position invites deep surrender, allowing the weight of your body to release into the support beneath you. The gentle movement of your lower back helps release deeply held tension while the open position of your legs allows constriction in the hips, where we often hold emotional stress, to gradually dissolve.

1. Lower yourself to lie on your back, feeling the support of the floor beneath your entire posterior body.
2. Bring the soles of your feet to touch, allowing your knees to fall outward like the opening of butterfly wings.
3. Position your arms alongside your body with palms facing upward in a gesture of receptivity.
4. Close your eyes to turn your attention inward, focusing on the rhythmic rising and falling of your breath in your abdomen.
5. Initiate a subtle rocking motion by gently pressing your lower back into the floor and then releasing it, creating a micro-movement that helps release deeply held tension.
6. Continue this subtle, releasing movement for 1-2 minutes, or if deeper restoration is needed, hold the static pose for 3-5 minutes, allowing gravity to facilitate your body's natural unwinding.

Meditation and Mindfulness Practices

More than just trendy terms, mindfulness and meditation are vital survival skills in a world that thrives on chaos. Think of them as your zen alarm system, helping you stay calm and in control even when life challenges you.

These exercises teach us how to find calm amid chaos, how to sit with discomfort without losing control, and how to be at peace with uncertainty. And once you start, you'll wonder why you didn't sign up for this sooner.

These techniques are all about observing—not engaging. You'll become a witness to your thoughts, not a participant. We're teaching ourselves to breathe through those moments of discomfort and not resist the rollercoaster of life. But let's be real: meditation isn't one-size-fits-all. There are a lot of methods out there, and each works it's kind of magic. Here are a few that tend to kick stress to the curb like a boss:

1. **Mindfulness Meditation:** It's all about now. Forget about tomorrow's to-do list or the drama from last week. With mindfulness meditation, you're zeroing in on the present—your breath, your body, whatever's happening right now. Think of it as hitting the pause button on a chaotic scene, where you can just observe without getting swept away. It's the skill of letting your thoughts drift by without holding on to them, much like clouds. Regular practice will help you become more self-aware, focus better, and experience less stress. It's a life improvement, to put it another way.

2. **Loving-Kindness Meditation (Metta):** Loving-kindness meditation is all about spreading those warm, fuzzy vibes—not just to others but also to yourself. This is where you send out all the love, kindness, and compassion, visualizing it expanding like a soft glow. You repeat phrases, focus on positive feelings, and nurture that sense of love. The real kicker here? It can soften the rough edges of negative emotions and boost your positivity.

3. **Body Scan Meditation:** For those who feel like stress is permanently lodged in their body (hello, neck and shoulders), body scan meditation is your new best friend. Starting from your toes, you slowly scan up through your body, paying attention to areas where tension is hanging out. The goal is to release that built-up stress, one body part at a time. Not only does this help you relax, but it also makes you more aware of how your body's holding onto tension (and how to let it go). If you're struggling with sleep or constantly holding tension in your body, this meditation method is a game-changer.

Mindfulness Meditation

1. Find a comfortable seated position—on a chair, cushion, or floor. Keep your back straight but relaxed.
2. Close your eyes or lower your gaze.
3. Take a few deep breaths, allowing yourself to settle into the present moment.
4. Bring your attention to your breath. Notice the sensation as it enters and leaves your body.
5. Let your breath flow naturally, focusing on the rise and fall of your abdomen or the feeling of air through your nostrils.
6. When (not if) your mind wanders, gently bring your focus back to the breath—no judgment, just awareness.
7. Start with 5-10 minutes, increasing the duration as you become more comfortable.
8. To end, slowly bring awareness back to your surroundings, wiggle your fingers and toes, and open your eyes.

Loving-Kindness Meditation (Metta)

1. Sit comfortably, close your eyes, and take a few deep breaths.
2. Focus on your heart center—imagine a warm, glowing light in your chest.
3. Silently repeat:

    - May I be happy.
    - May I be healthy.
    - May I be safe.
    - May I live with ease.

1. After a few minutes, bring to mind someone you care deeply about and offer them the same wishes:

    - May you be happy.
    - May you be healthy.
    - May you be safe.
    - May you live with ease.

2. Next, extend this to a neutral person—someone you neither like nor dislike.

3. If you feel ready, offer these wishes to someone you struggle with.
4. Finally, expand your intention to all beings everywhere.
5. Practice for 10-15 minutes, then gently return to your surroundings.

Body Scan Meditation

1. Lie down in a comfortable position, arms at your sides, palms facing up.
2. Close your eyes and take a few deep breaths to relax.
3. Begin at your toes, noticing any sensations—warmth, tingling, tension, or numbness.
4. Slowly move upward, scanning your body part by part:

    - Feet → Ankles → Calves → Knees → Thighs
    - Hips → Lower back → Abdomen → Chest
    - Upper back → Fingers → Hands → Arms → Shoulders
    - Neck → Jaw → Head

5. If you feel tension in any area, breathe into it and imagine it softening.
6. If your mind drifts, gently bring it back to the body part you're focusing on.
7. Once you've scanned your entire body, take a moment to feel your body as a whole.
8. To end, wiggle your fingers and toes, take a deep breath, and open your eyes.
9. Start with 10-15 minutes, increasing the duration as needed.

Chapter 6: Tension Release and Trauma Management Exercises

Trauma is not what happens to you, it's what happens inside you as a result of what happened to you.—Gabor Maté

I had a conversation with a somatic therapist recently that completely shifted my perspective. We were talking about healing, and she hit me with this powerful insight: "You can't heal in the same environments that made you sick." That statement stuck with me because it didn't just apply to physical spaces. It spoke to something deeper. "Environment" isn't just about your external surroundings—it's the internal landscape we carry around: our thoughts, our reactions, the tension in our muscles, the rhythms of our breath. The stories and patterns we've picked up from past experiences, especially trauma, shape this internal environment. These mental and physical states can keep us trapped in cycles of stress and pain long after the original events have passed.

Healing happens when we reshape this internal landscape. The key is to transform the way we respond to life through mindful movement, awareness, and practices that help us break free from the cycles of trauma. Every time you step into that space of mindful awareness, remember: you're laying down new neural pathways. You're teaching your body how to be different—so much so that healing becomes not just possible but inevitable. It's like creating a new home for yourself inside your own body—a space where safety, peace, and release are the foundation.

Why Tension Occurs

Tension is your body's natural defense mechanism. It's that physical and emotional strain we feel when we're stressed, facing a threat, or dealing with something challenging. Stress activates the nervous system, triggering muscle contraction, quickening the heart rate, and heightening alertness. This is a protective response, preparing us for action when danger seems near.

However, when trauma strikes—especially if it's severe or prolonged—this fight-or-flight response doesn't always have the chance to dissipate. The body goes into a hyper-alert state, and if we don't fully process or release the experience, that heightened stress can stick around. It's like the body's "protective armor" that never takes off. Tension accumulates and becomes chronic. This means tight muscles, shallow breathing, and an overactive nervous system.

And it doesn't stop there. Chronic tension can lead to a whole series of physical and psychological challenges. Pain, reduced flexibility, and structural imbalances show up, not to mention the emotional toll—anxiety, irritability, and a general inability to relax. It's a vicious cycle that makes it harder to fully experience the present moment because part of your energy is always dedicated to maintaining that state of "alert readiness." Eventually, the nervous system gets so dysregulated that returning to a state of calm feels nearly impossible.

Symptoms of Tension

Tension doesn't have a one-size-fits-all appearance—it shows up differently depending on where it's hanging out in your body and mind. Here are some telltale signs that you might be carrying around more tension than you'd like:

Physical Symptoms:

1. Muscle tightness or stiffness, especially in the neck, shoulders, and back
2. Headaches, particularly tension headaches
3. Jaw-clenching or teeth-grinding
4. Chest tightness
5. Rapid heartbeat
6. Shallow or rapid breathing
7. Digestive issues (e.g., stomachaches, nausea, constipation, or diarrhea)
8. Fatigue or low-energy
9. Insomnia or disturbed sleep
10. Sweating, especially in the palms or armpits
11. Cold hands or feet
12. Frequent urination
13. Decreased libido

Emotional Symptoms:

1. Irritability or short temper
2. Anxiety or nervousness

3. Mood swings
4. Feeling overwhelmed
5. Depression or persistent low mood
6. Emotional numbness
7. Increased emotional reactivity
8. Difficulty feeling joy or pleasure

Cognitive Symptoms:

1. Difficulty concentrating or focusing
2. Racing thoughts
3. Forgetfulness or memory problems
4. Indecisiveness
5. Constant worrying
6. Negative self-talk
7. Difficulty in problem-solving
8. Decreased creativity

Behavioral Symptoms:

1. Procrastination or avoiding responsibilities
2. Nervous habits (e.g., nail biting, hair twirling, foot tapping)
3. Changes in appetite (eating too much or too little)
4. Increased use of alcohol, cigarettes, or drugs
5. Social withdrawal
6. Relationship conflicts
7. Decreased productivity
8. Restlessness or inability to relax

Everyone experiences tension differently, and you may not have all these symptoms. However, if several of them persist, it could indicate significant tension. In such cases, incorporating tension-release exercises, seeking support from a mental health professional, or consulting a healthcare provider can be beneficial.

SOMATIC EXERCISES FOR NERVOUS SYSTEM REGULATION

Somatic Movement for Tension Release

Seated Forward Fold with Rocking

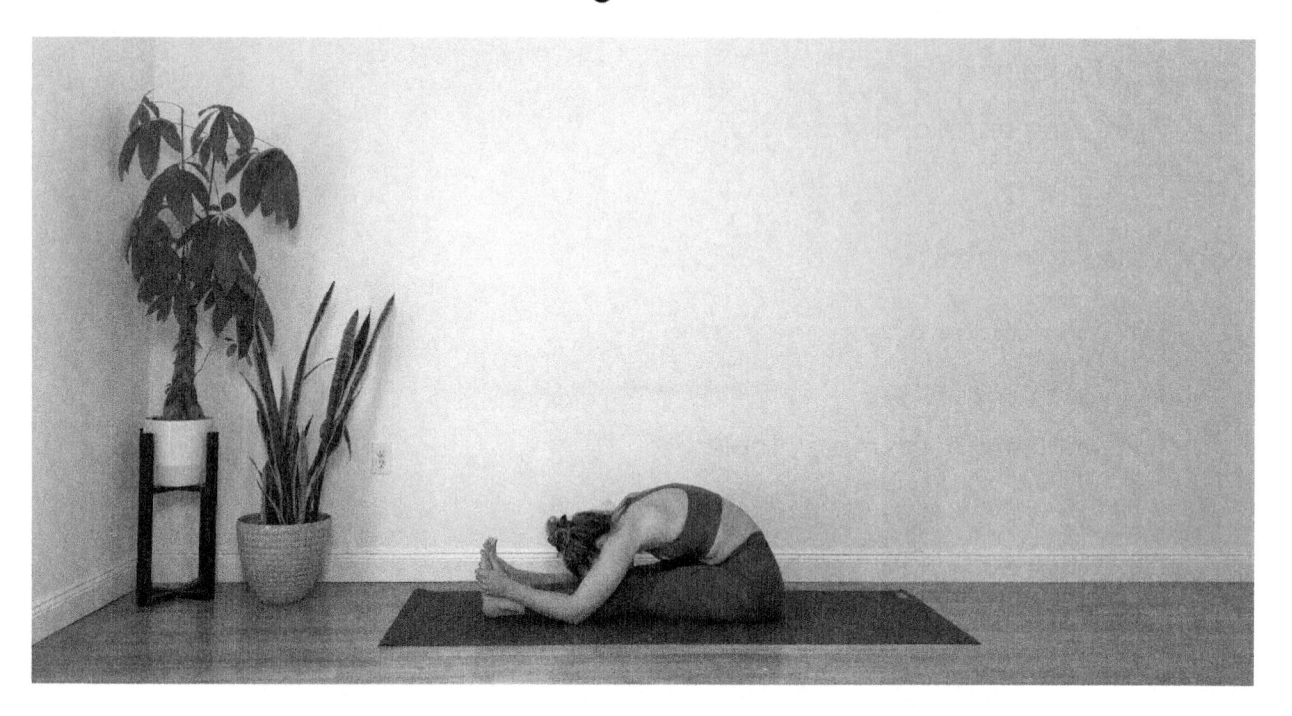

This gentle forward fold invites you to surrender the weight of your day through your spine, an area where we unconsciously store the tensions of our experiences. The rhythmic rocking motion helps release layers of holding that have become embedded in the back body, creating a sense of both freedom and grounding.

1. Find a comfortable seated position with your legs extended forward, creating a foundation of support.

2. Draw a deep breath in, allowing your spine to grow tall as if being gently pulled upward.

3. As you release your breath, initiate a mindful folding from your hip creases, sending your heart forward toward your feet.

4. Allow your upper body to surrender its weight, your head hanging heavy as tension begins to dissolve.

5. Begin a gentle, rhythmic rocking motion forward and back, noticing how the sensation shifts through different areas of your back with each movement.

6. Continue this soothing, wavelike motion for 30-60 seconds, synchronizing with your natural breathing rhythm.

7. When ready to return, slowly stack your spine one vertebra at a time, honoring the renewed spaciousness you've created.

Thread The Needle

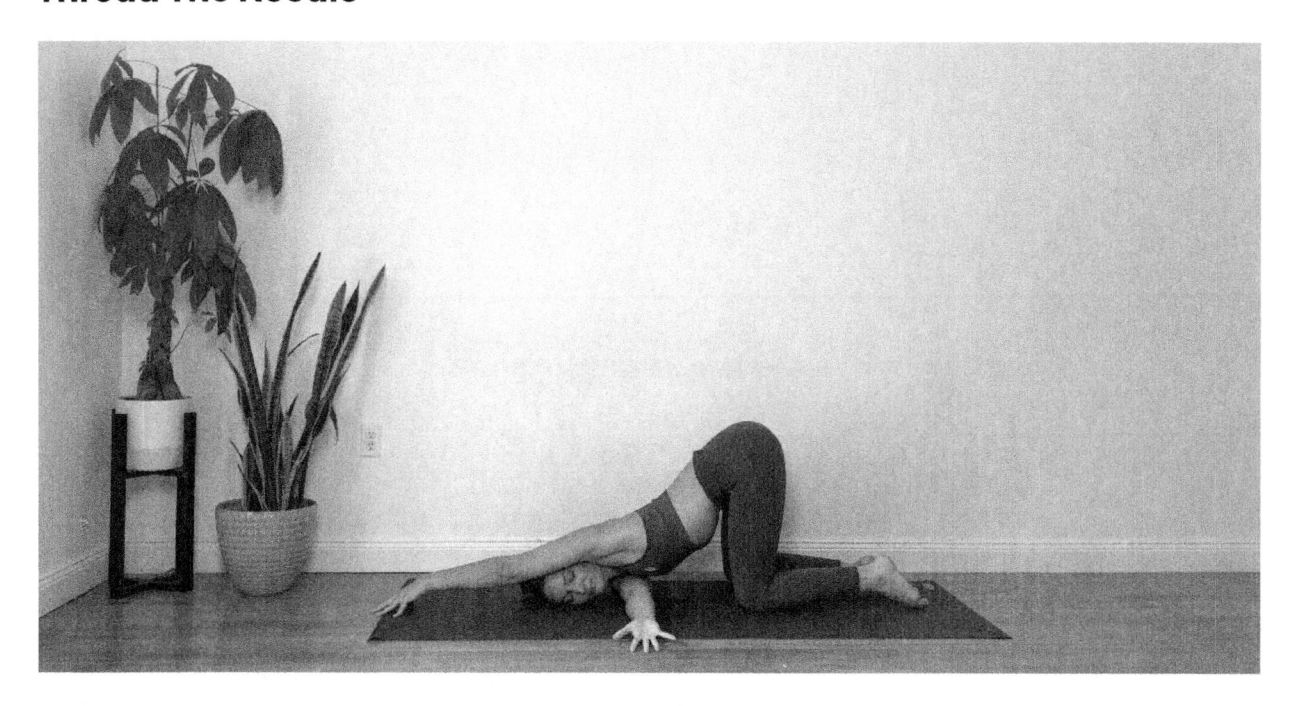

This profound twist offers release for the spaces between your shoulder blades, an area where we often hold the burden of responsibilities unaddressed. By creating this unusual position, you're inviting your nervous system to let go of familiar patterns and discover new possibilities for freedom in your upper body.

1. Begin in a tabletop position, creating a stable foundation with your hands and knees.
2. Slide your right arm underneath your left arm and through the opening between your left arm and knee as if threading an invisible needle.
3. Allow your right shoulder and the side of your head to melt toward the earth, surrendering to gravity.
4. Keep your left hand planted for stability, or if your body invites a deeper experience, extend it forward to create additional length.
5. Remain in this releasing position for 30 seconds to 1 minute, allowing each breath to soften areas of resistance.
6. Mindfully unwind back to your starting position, noticing the contrast between the two sides of your body.
7. Honor the other side by threading your left arm under your right, creating balance in your practice.
8. Complete 2-3 rounds on each side, allowing each repetition to access deeper layers of release.

Seated Side Bend

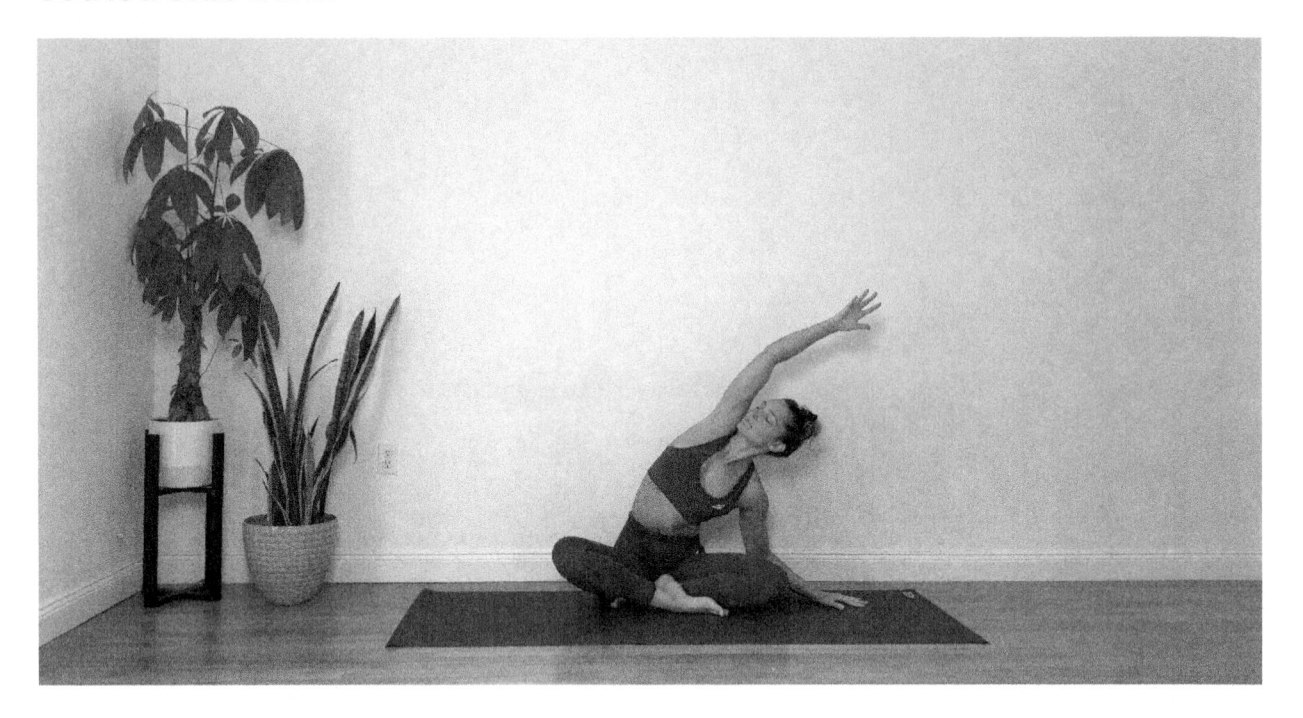

The sides of our bodies often become forgotten territories, compressed by daily activities and emotional holding. This mindful lateral stretch creates space between each rib, allowing for fuller breath and releasing constriction in these overlooked areas that connect our upper and lower body.

1. Find a comfortable seated position, either with legs crossed or extended, based on what feels supportive for your body.
2. Extend your right arm skyward while your left hand rests on the floor to provide stability and support.
3. Draw a full breath in, feeling how this action creates natural length along your right side.
4. As you exhale, initiate a gentle lateral curve to the left, creating space between each rib on your right side.
5. Remain here for 3-5 breath cycles, noticing how your ribcage expands and contracts with each breath.
6. Mindfully return to the center before honoring the opposite side with the same attentive movement.
7. Complete 3-5 side bends on each side, approaching each repetition with renewed awareness rather than mechanical repetition.

CHAPTER 6: TENSION RELEASE AND TRAUMA MANAGEMENT EXERCISES

Seated Figure Four Stretch

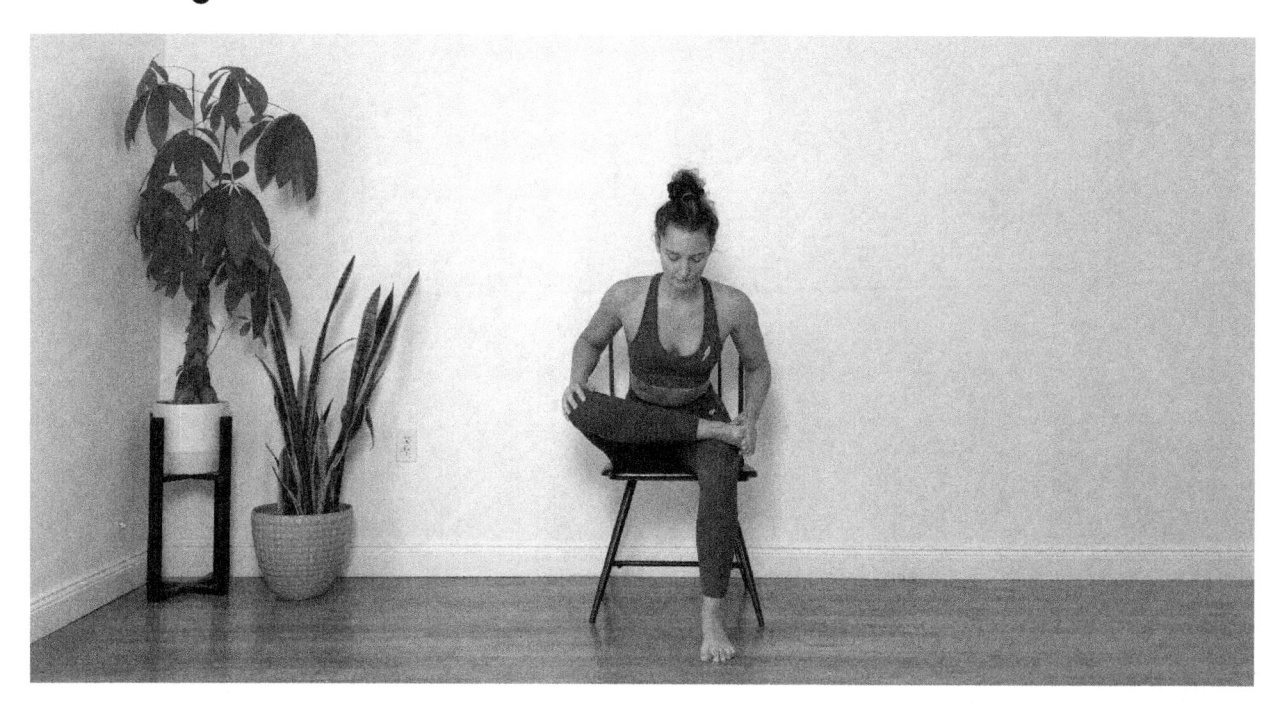

The hips cradle unprocessed emotions and stress, often becoming repositories for tension we've not had space to acknowledge. This gentle opening, combined with soothing movement, helps release both physical restriction and the emotional residue that accompanies it.

1. Sit toward the edge of your chair, allowing both feet to make solid contact with the floor.
2. Cross your right ankle over your left thigh, creating a figure-four shape that begins to open the outer hip.
3. Activate your right foot by flexing it, creating a protective engagement that safeguards your knee.
4. Grow tall through your spine, imagining a thread drawing upward from the crown of your head.
5. Initiate a gentle hinging forward from your hip creases, exploring the sensation of opening in your right hip.
6. Begin a subtle, rhythmic rocking motion, moving slightly forward and back, helping to release layers of held tension.
7. Continue this soothing movement for 30-60 seconds, allowing your breath to remain steady and full.
8. Mindfully transition to the opposite side, noticing any differences between your right and left hips.

SOMATIC EXERCISES FOR NERVOUS SYSTEM REGULATION

Seated Arm Circles

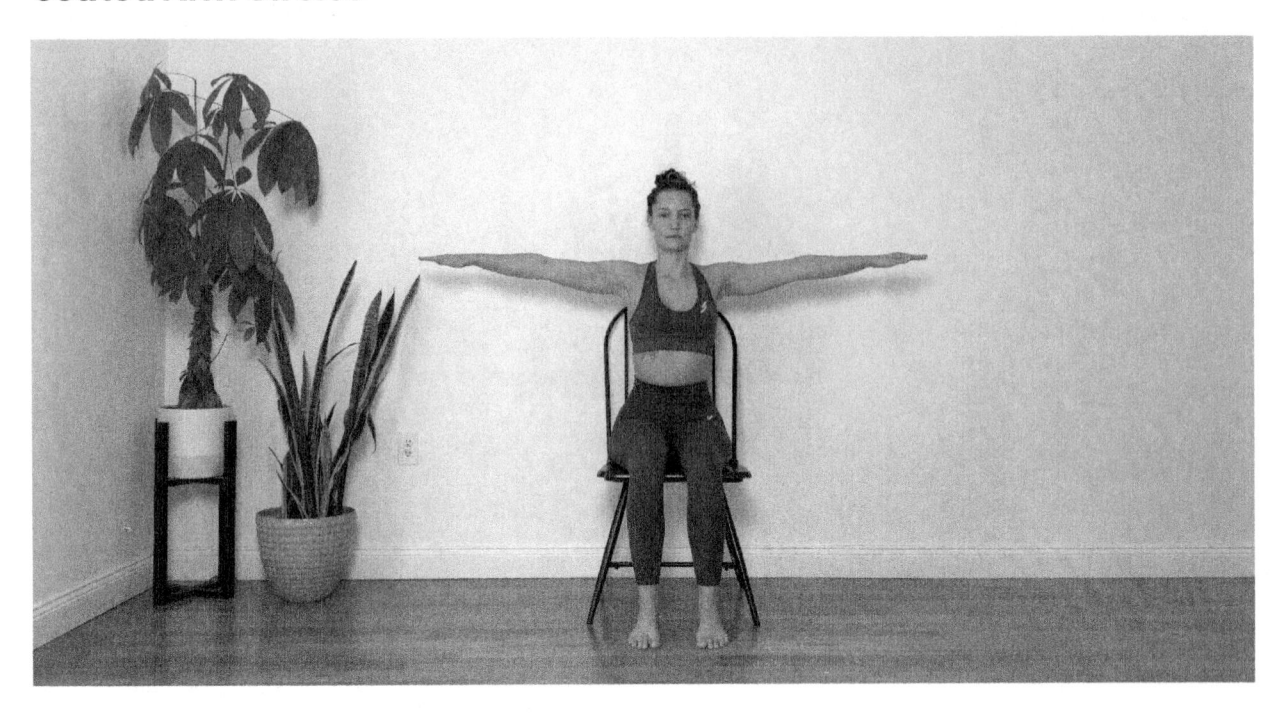

The shoulders often carry the weight of both physical and emotional burdens, becoming repositories for tension that goes unaddressed. These flowing circles help release what's been stored in your upper body, creating freedom where restriction has become the norm.

1. Sit with your spine naturally aligned, feet making grounded contact with the floor beneath you.
2. Extend your arms outward from your shoulders, creating a T-shape with your upper body.
3. Initiate small, mindful circular motions with your arms, noticing the subtle sensations this creates throughout your shoulder complex.
4. Gradually allow the circles to expand, always staying within the range that feels nourishing rather than straining.
5. After 30 seconds of this unwinding movement, reverse the direction, noticing how this simple change creates new awareness.
6. Bring your attention to your breathing pattern and the changing sensations throughout your shoulders, arms, and upper back.
7. Continue this rhythmic exploration for 1-2 minutes, allowing the movement to help dissolve accumulated tension.

Somatic Chest Opener

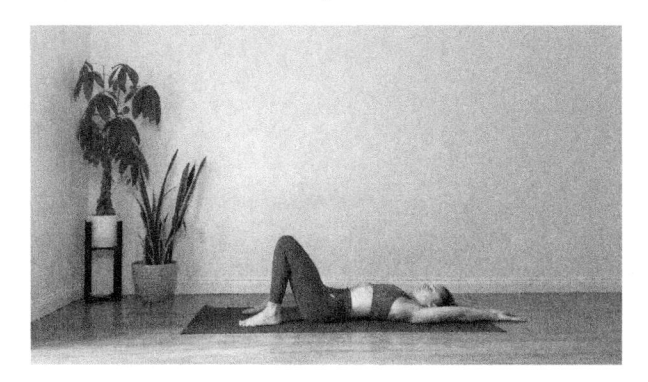

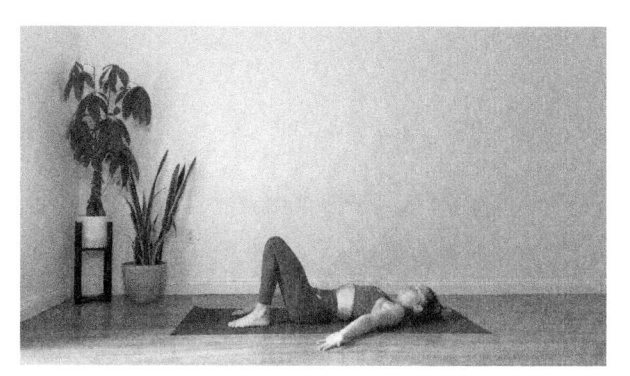

The chest often becomes constricted by both physical habits and emotional guardedness. This gentle opening creates space for fuller breath and helps release the armor we unconsciously build around our hearts, allowing for a more authentic connection with ourselves and others.

1. Lower yourself to lie on your back, knees bent with feet planted firmly on the floor for support.
2. Extend your arms out to your sides with palms facing upward in a gesture of receptivity.
3. Draw a deep, nourishing breath in, feeling how your chest naturally expands with this action.
4. As you exhale, create a gentle grounding by pressing your arms into the supporting surface beneath you.
5. Initiate a slow, mindful movement of your arms upward toward your head, then back down alongside your body.
6. Bring your awareness to the opening sensation across your chest and the subtle movement of your shoulder blades against the floor.
7. Repeat this flowing movement 5-10 times, moving at a pace that allows you to notice the subtleties of sensation rather than rushing through the exercise.

Reclined Hamstring Stretch

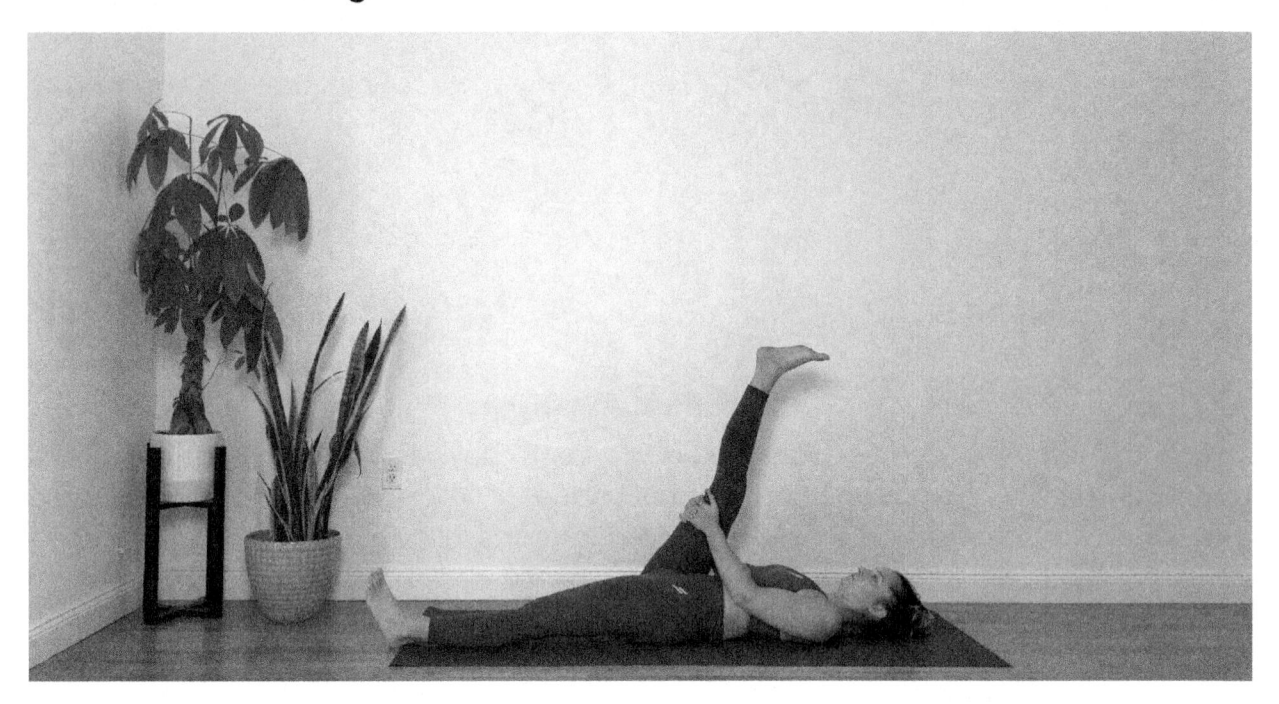

The hamstrings often hold the tension of our busy lives, becoming shortened and tight as we move through our days. This supine position allows for both support and surrender, helping these powerful muscles release their habitual holding patterns while calming your nervous system.

1. Lie back with both legs extended, allowing your entire back body to be supported by the floor beneath you.
2. Mindfully lift your right leg toward the ceiling, maintaining a slight bend in the knee if needed.
3. Support this position by placing your hands behind your thigh, or use a strap around your foot if this feels more accessible for your body.
4. Explore the changing sensations by alternately flexing and pointing your foot, noticing how this simple movement affects the entire back of your leg.
5. Introduce gentle circles with your ankle in both directions, helping to release tension throughout the entire leg.
6. Remain here for 30-60 seconds, breathing deeply into any areas of resistance or holding.
7. With mindfulness, lower your leg and repeat this nurturing stretch with your left leg.

CHAPTER 6: TENSION RELEASE AND TRAUMA MANAGEMENT EXERCISES

Somatic Frog Pose

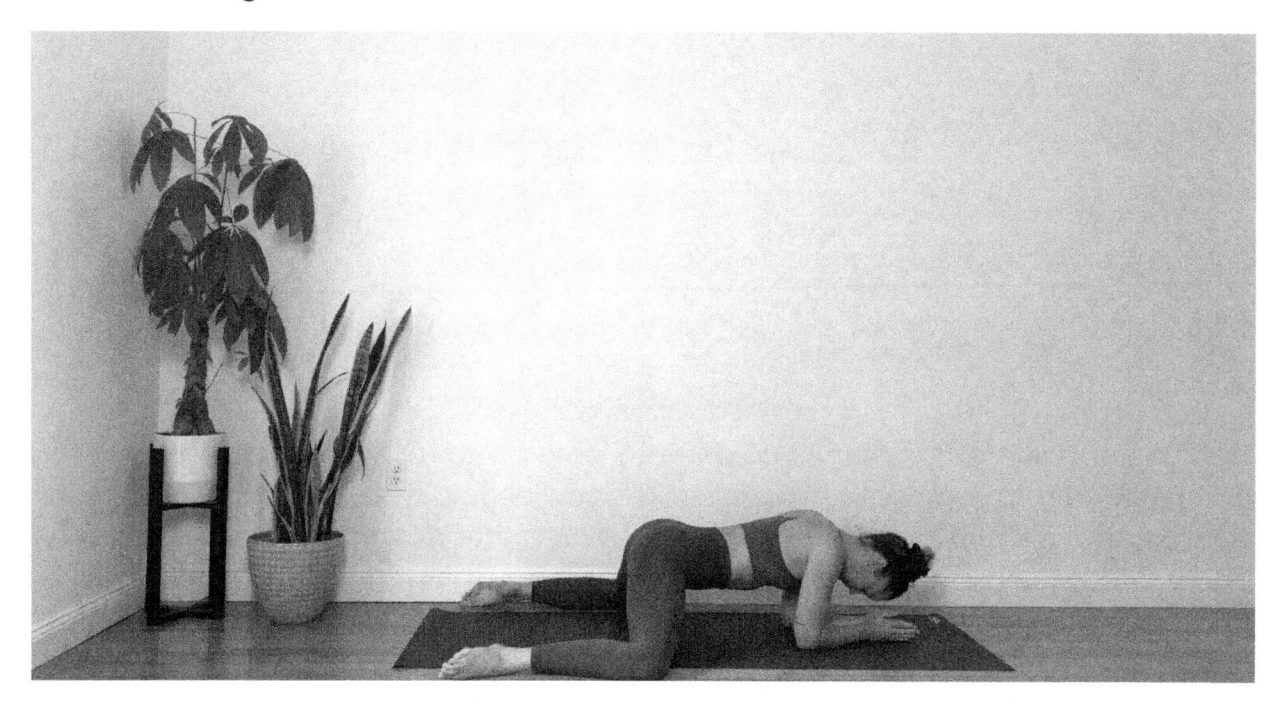

The hips store the residue of our daily stresses and unexpressed emotions. This supported opening, combined with gentle movement, helps release deeply held patterns and creates new space in an area that profoundly affects our overall freedom of movement and emotional well-being.

1. Begin in a tabletop position, creating a stable foundation with your hands and knees.

2. Gradually widen your knees apart while keeping your feet in proximity to each other, honoring your body's current range.

3. Lower your upper body onto your forearms, creating a supportive base that allows your hips to release more fully.

4. Initiate a gentle, rhythmic rocking motion with your hips, moving them slightly forward and back.

5. Bring your awareness to your breath and the changing sensations throughout your inner thighs and hips as you continue this movement.

6. Sustain this unwinding motion for 30-60 seconds, allowing each movement to access deeper layers of release.

7. With mindfulness, return to the tabletop position, noticing the renewed sensation of space and freedom in your lower body.

SOMATIC EXERCISES FOR NERVOUS SYSTEM REGULATION

Somatic Cobra Pose

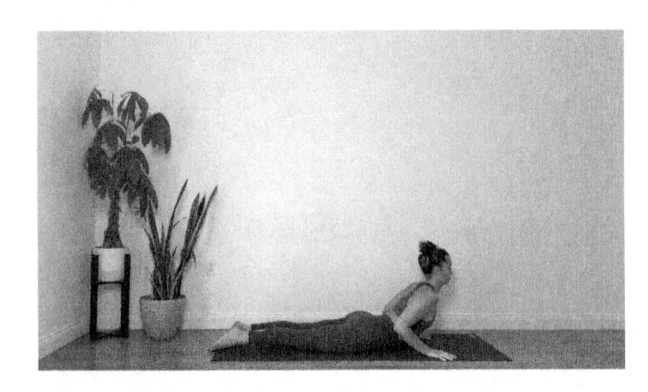

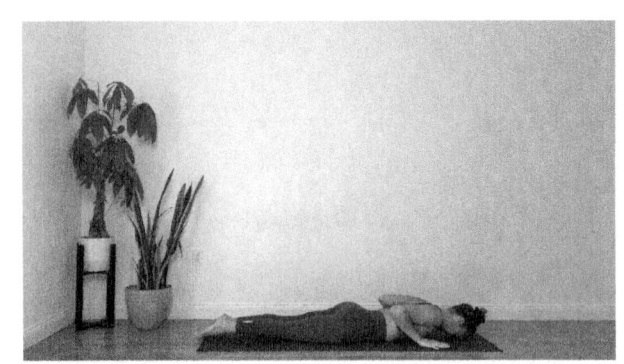

This gentle backbend invites your spine to emerge from its protective curling, an instinctive pattern we adopt when facing life's challenges. By initiating movement from your upper back, you're reconnecting with an area that often becomes rigid through daily activities and emotional holding.

1. Rest face down, allowing your forehead to release onto the floor and positioning your hands alongside your shoulders.

2. As you draw breath in, initiate a gentle lifting of your chest away from the earth, keeping your lower body soft and receptive.

3. With your exhale, slowly return to the ground, surrendering any unnecessary tension.

4. Bring your awareness to initiating this movement from your upper back rather than pushing with your hands.

5. Continue this mindful undulation 5-10 times, noticing how each repetition may allow for new freedom.

6. Move with deliberate slowness, allowing each breath to guide the timing of your movement.

CHAPTER 6: TENSION RELEASE AND TRAUMA MANAGEMENT EXERCISES

Somatic Half-Bow Pose

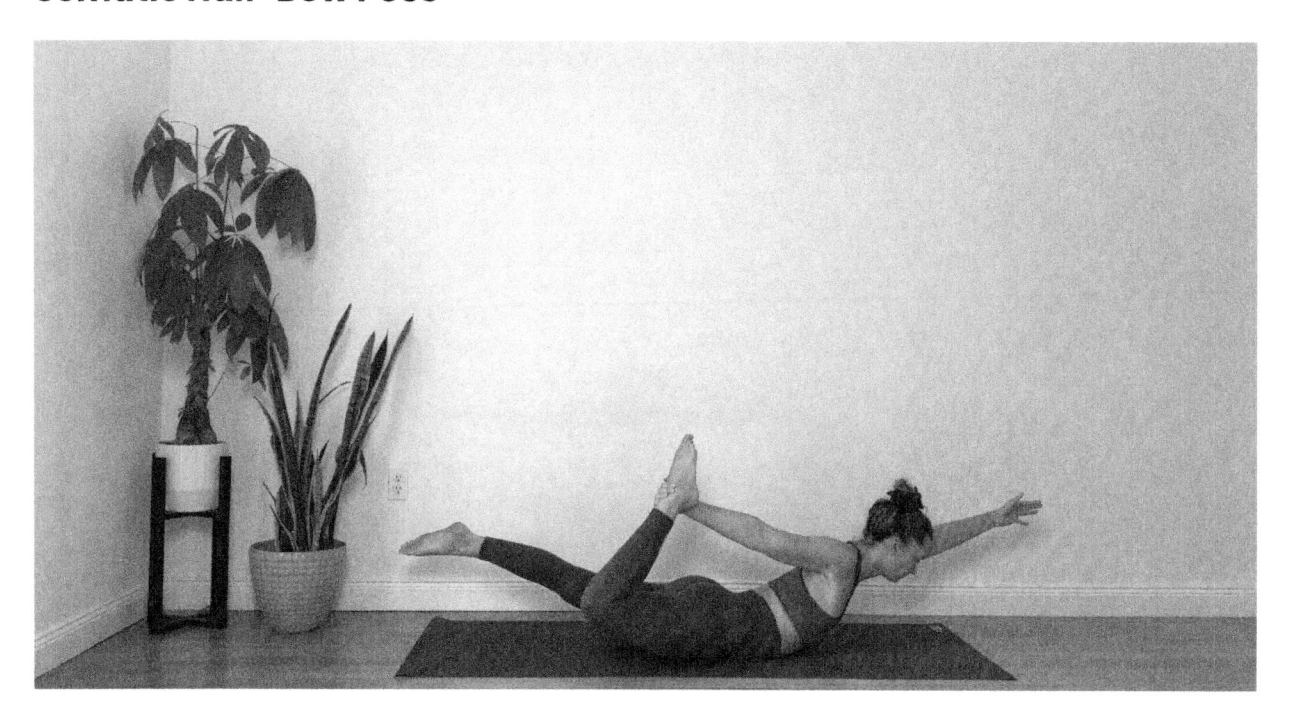

The front of the body often becomes compressed through protective posturing and habitual patterns. This exercise creates a gentle opening across the chest and hip flexors, areas where we store the residue of stress responses and emotional holding.

1. Allow your body to rest face down, with arms resting naturally alongside your torso.
2. Bend your right knee, guiding your heel in the direction of your sitting bones.
3. With mindfulness, reach back with your right hand to make a gentle connection with your right ankle.
4. As you inhale, initiate a subtle lifting of your right leg away from the floor, creating a gentle opening across the front of your hip and thigh.
5. With your exhale, release back to the earth, surrendering any unnecessary effort.
6. Repeat this nurturing movement 5-7 times, each repetition an opportunity for deeper release.
7. Mindfully release this position before honoring the left side with the same attentive movement.

Child's Pose with Arm Walks

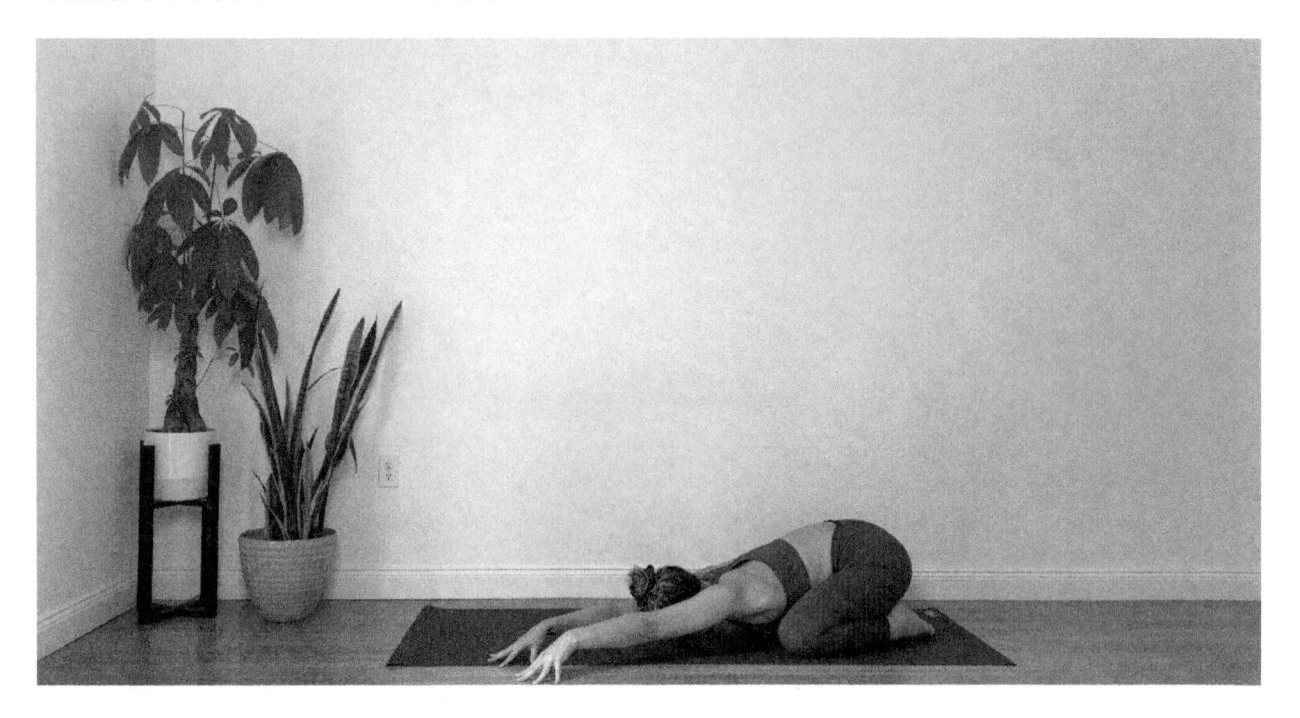

Child's Pose offers a return to safety and surrender, while the arm walks create gentle lateral stretching that helps release tension held in the spaces between the ribs. This combination promotes both grounding and freedom in areas often constricted by stress.

Find your way into Child's Pose, knees comfortably widened with big toes touching, creating a secure base.

1. Extend your arms forward along the floor, establishing length through your spine.
2. Begin walking your hands to the right, inviting a gentle stretch to spread along the left side of the body.
3. Remain here for 3-5 complete breath cycles, allowing each exhale to release deeper layers of tension.
4. With mindfulness, guide your hands back to the center before initiating the same movement toward the left.
5. Honor this side with 3-5 full breaths, noticing any differences between the right and left sides of your body.
6. Continue this balancing sequence 3-5 times on each side, allowing each repetition to access new awareness.

Somatic Scapula Mobilization

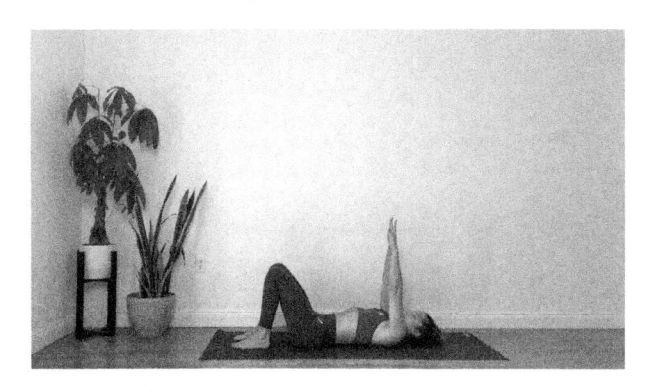

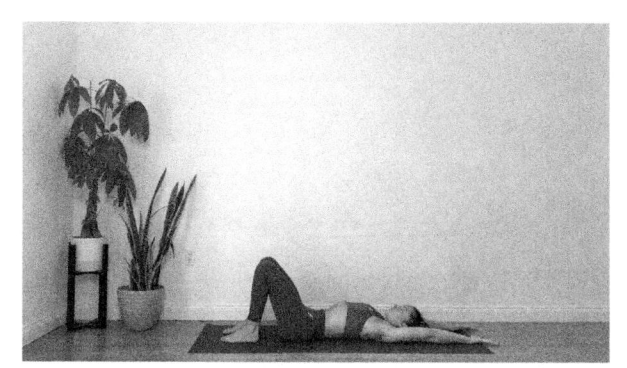

1. The shoulder blades often become restricted through daily activities and emotional holding. This exercise invites freedom in an area critical for healthy arm movement and upper body release, helping to dissolve patterns of tension that affect both posture and breathing.

2. Settle onto your back, knees bent with feet establishing a solid connection to the floor.

3. Extend your arms toward the ceiling, creating length without tension.

4. Initiate a slow reaching movement upward and back, as if your fingertips are drawn toward a point beyond your head.

5. Then, guide your arms in the opposite direction, moving toward your hips with the same mindful attention.

6. Bring your awareness to the subtle movements of your shoulder blades against the floor as they glide with each motion.

7. Continue this flowing exploration 10-15 times, moving at a pace that allows you to notice the subtleties rather than rushing through the exercise.

Somatic Pigeon Pose

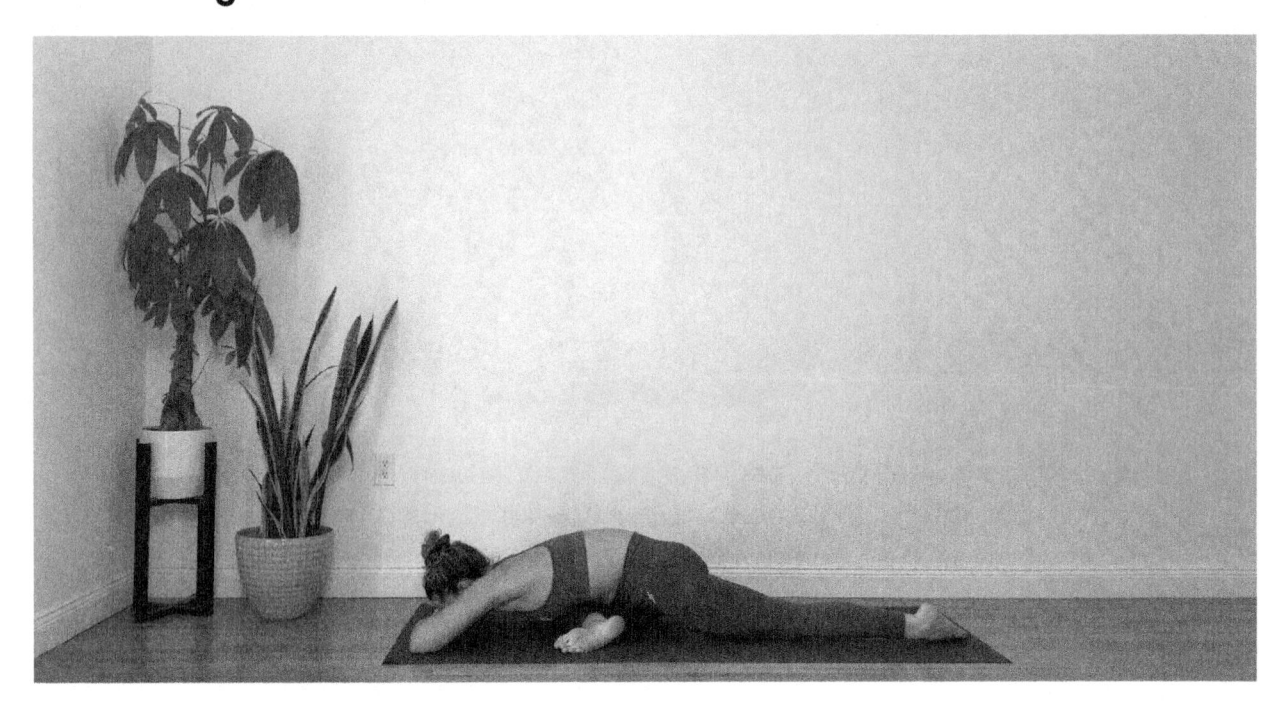

The hips cradle unprocessed emotions and stress, often becoming repositories for tension we've not had space to acknowledge. The gentle rocking motion helps release both physical restriction and the emotional residue that accompanies it, creating new freedom for both body and mind.

1. Begin in a tabletop position, creating a stable foundation with your hands and knees.
2. Guide your right knee forward, placing it behind your right wrist while maintaining awareness of your knee's comfort.
3. Extend your left leg behind you, creating length from hip to heel.
4. Lower your upper body onto your forearms or allow your forehead to make contact with the floor, surrendering to gravity.
5. Initiate a gentle side-to-side rocking motion with your hips, helping to release layers of held tension.
6. Bring your awareness to your breath and the changing sensations throughout your right hip as you continue this movement.
7. Sustain this unwinding motion for 30-60 seconds, allowing each movement to access deeper layers of release.
8. With mindfulness, return to the tabletop before honoring the left hip with the same nurturing attention.

Reclined Spinal Twist

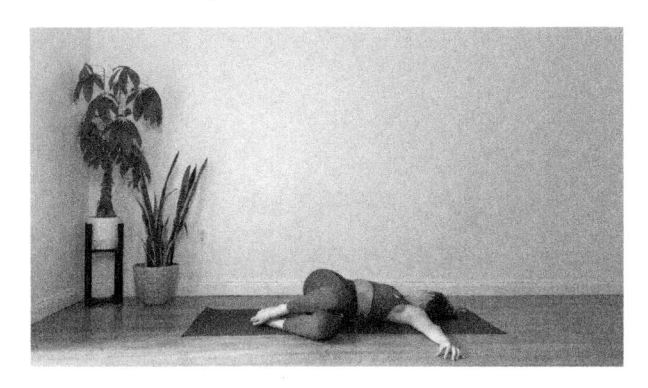

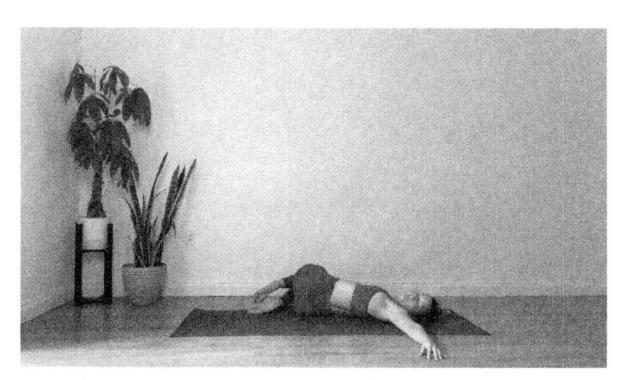

Twisting movements help unwind the accumulated tension that builds between the vertebrae through daily activities and stress responses. This gentle rotation creates space and releases holding patterns that can restrict both movement and breath.

1. Lie on your back, knees drawn toward your chest and feet lifted to create a 90-degree angle at your knees.

2. Extend your arms outward to form a T-shape with your torso, creating stability through your upper body.

3. While maintaining the grounding of your shoulders, guide both knees to lower toward the right side of your body.

4. If it feels nourishing, turn your head to the left, creating a gentle counterrotation through your spine.

5. Remain here for 5-10 full breath cycles, allowing each exhale to invite a deeper release through your spine and hips.

6. With your next inhale, mindfully guide your knees back to center, acknowledging the sensations this movement creates.

7. Continue by lowering your knees to the left side, honoring both sides of your body with equal attention.

Dynamic Bridge Pose

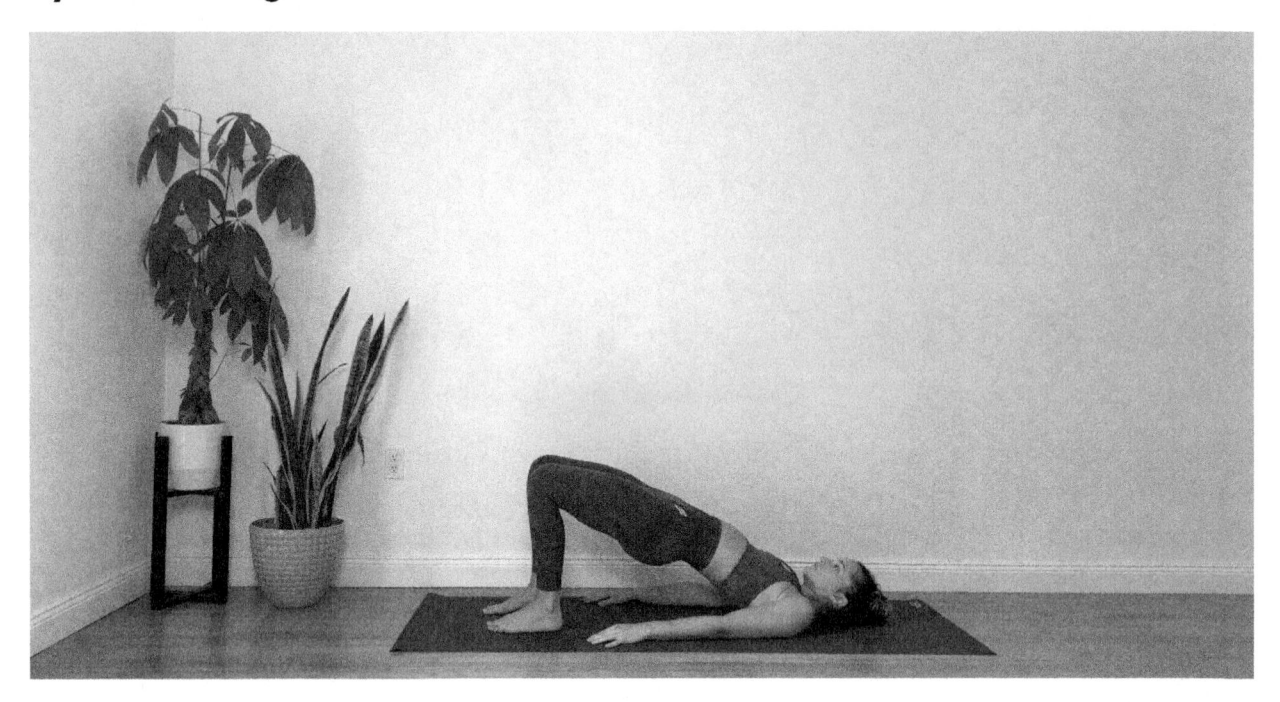

This flowing movement creates a dialogue between stability and mobility in your spine. By rolling up and down through each vertebra, you're releasing deeply held tension while awakening awareness in areas that may have become rigid or numb through habitual patterns.

1. Lie down on your back, knees bent with feet planted firmly on the floor at hip-width distance.
2. Allow your arms to rest alongside your body, palms connecting with the floor to provide additional support.
3. As you inhale, initiate a slow rolling up through your spine, beginning with your tailbone and allowing each vertebra to lift sequentially.
4. With your exhale, reverse this mindful unraveling, descending through your spine one vertebra at a time.
5. Bring your awareness to the process of moving each segment of your spine individually rather than as a single unit.
6. Continue this wave-like movement 10-15 times, allowing your breath to naturally guide the timing of each undulation.

CHAPTER 6: TENSION RELEASE AND TRAUMA MANAGEMENT EXERCISES

Standing Spinal Wave

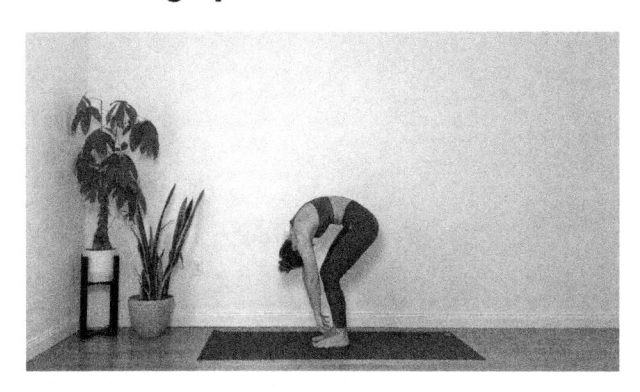

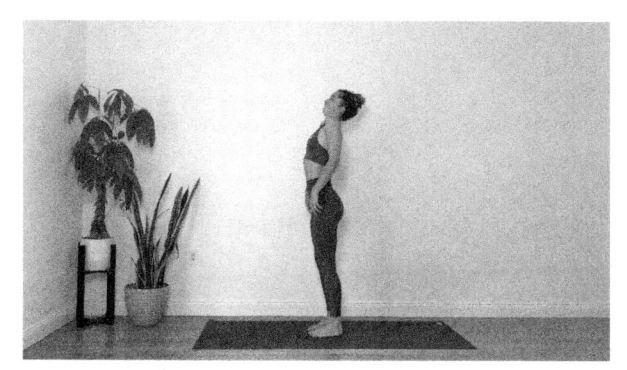

The spine houses not only our nervous system but also holds the residue of unexpressed emotions and stress. This flowing wave helps unwind the accumulated tension while promoting the healthy mobility that allows energy to flow more freely throughout your entire being.

1. Stand with your feet hip-width apart, knees slightly softened to remove unnecessary tension.
2. Begin by releasing your chin toward your chest, then continue this surrender through each vertebra, allowing gravity to assist.
3. When your forward fold is complete, pause briefly, allowing your upper body to hang heavy as tension begins to dissolve.
4. Initiate a mindful rolling up by engaging your deepest core muscles, stacking each vertebra with conscious awareness.
5. Once vertical, create a gentle arching through your spine, allowing your heart to lift and expand.
6. From this place of openness, begin the wave again by releasing your chin toward your chest.
7. Continue this fluid, wavelike motion for 1-2 minutes, noticing how each repetition may offer new freedom.
8. Synchronize your breath with this movement—exhale as you surrender downward, inhaling as you rise with intention.

Somatic Shoulder Bridge

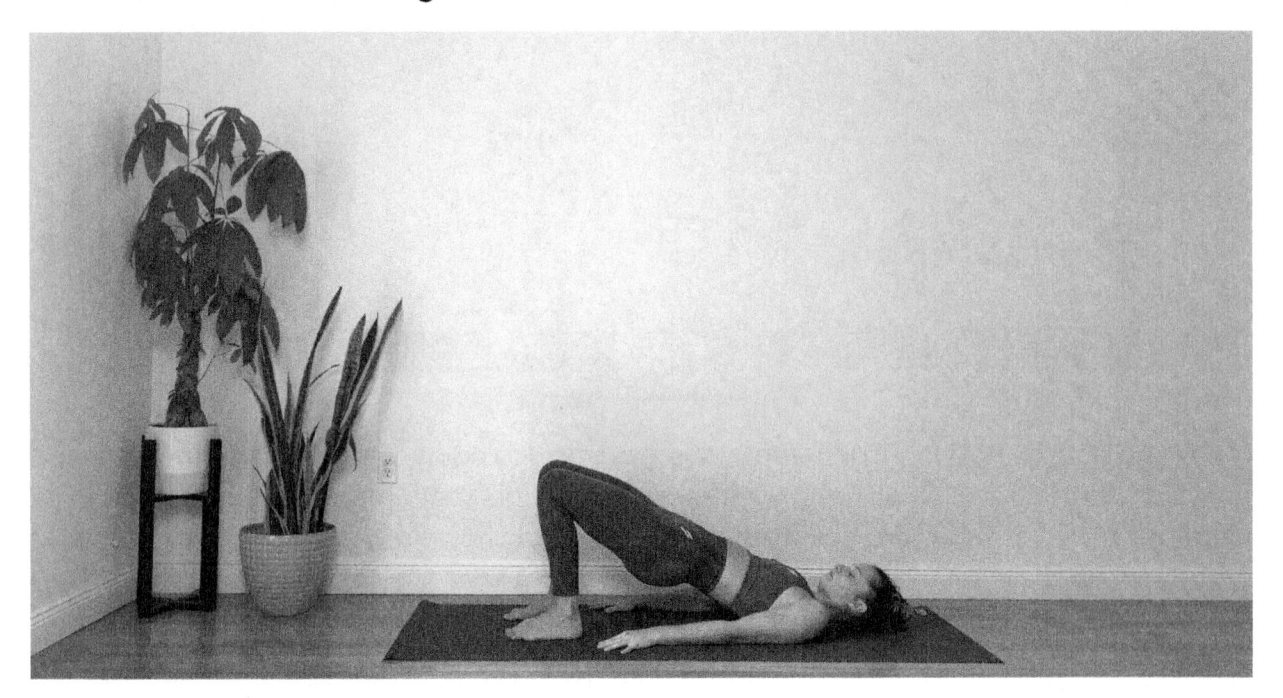

This movement creates a dialogue between stability and mobility in your spine and hips. By mindfully lifting and lowering, you're releasing tension in areas often held rigid while strengthening the supportive muscles that help maintain healthy alignment in daily life.

1. Rest on your back, knees bent with feet establishing a solid connection to the floor at hip-width distance.
2. Press your arms and shoulders deliberately into the floor, creating a stable foundation for movement.
3. As you inhale, initiate a mindful lifting of your hips away from the floor, creating a diagonal line of energy from knees to shoulders.
4. With your exhale, begin a controlled lowering, allowing each vertebra to make contact with the floor sequentially.
5. Bring your awareness to the process of moving each segment of your spine individually rather than as a single rigid unit.
6. Continue this deliberate movement 10-15 times, allowing your breath to naturally guide the timing of each repetition.

Knees to Chest Rocking

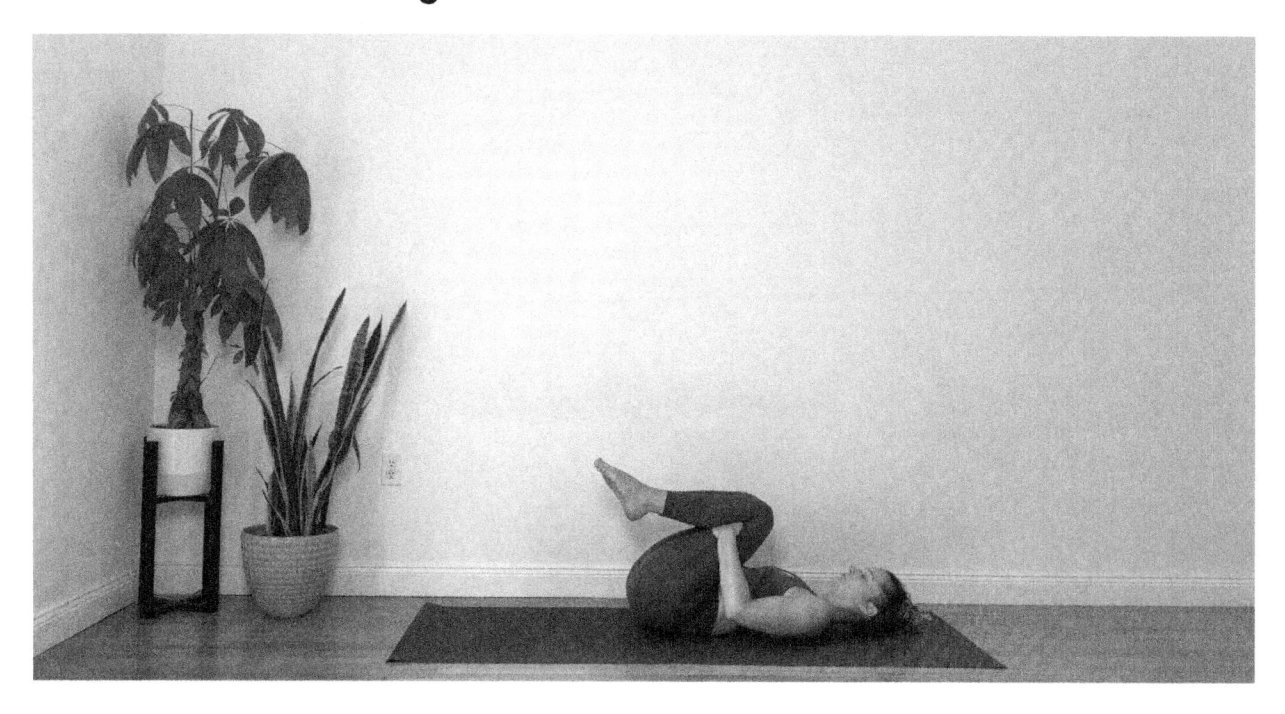

This gentle rocking motion helps release tension held in the lower back, an area where we often store stress and unprocessed emotions. The rhythmic movement provides a subtle massage for tight muscles while calming your nervous system.

Lie on your back and draw your knees toward your chest, creating a natural curve in your lower back.

1. Encircle your legs with your arms, either wrapped around your shins or supporting behind your thighs.
2. Initiate a gentle side-to-side rocking motion, allowing the floor to provide a subtle massage to your lower back muscles.
3. Bring your awareness to the changing sensations along your spine with each rocking movement.
4. Continue this soothing motion for 30-60 seconds, allowing your breath to remain deep and nourishing.

Supine Knee-to-Chest Pose (Apanasana)

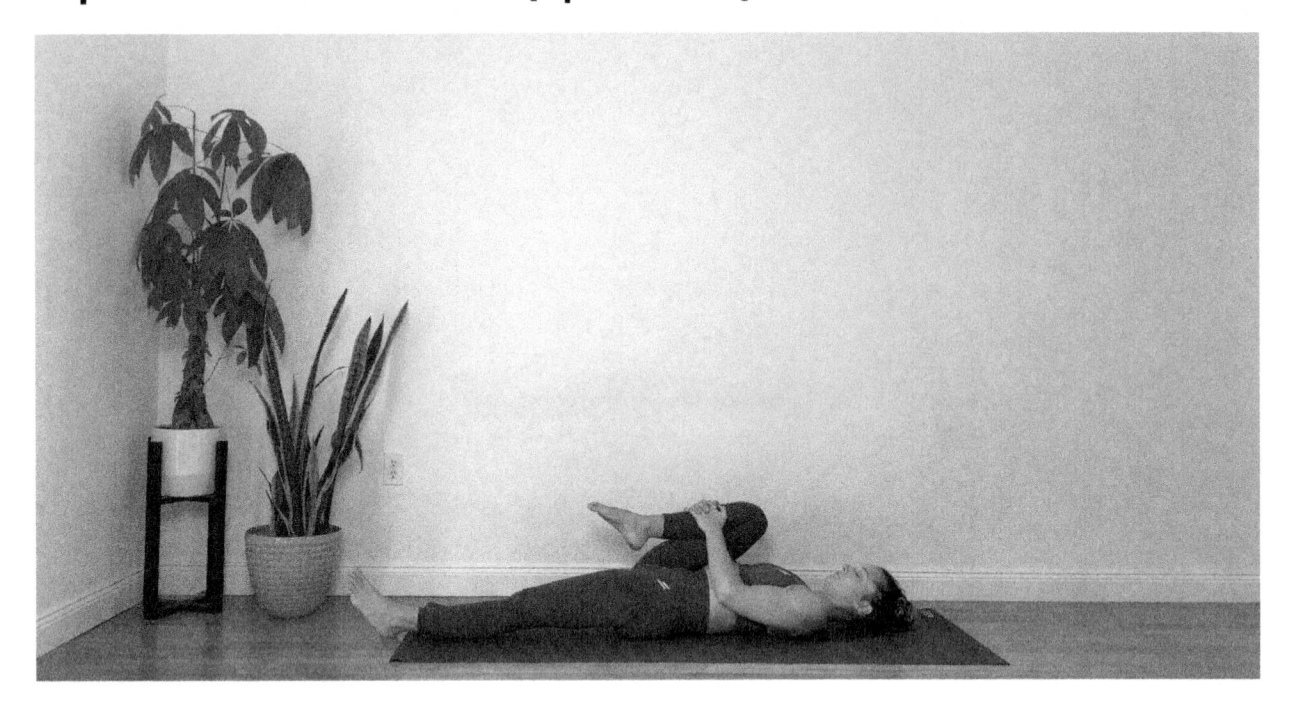

This nurturing pose helps release tension in the lower back and hips while creating gentle compression that supports digestive health. By working with one leg at a time, you're able to notice subtle imbalances that may exist between the two sides of your body.

1. Lie down on your back with your knees bent and feet making solid contact with the floor beneath you.

2. Draw your right knee toward your chest, holding it with both hands to create a gentle compression.

3. Either maintain your left foot on the floor or extend your left leg if this feels more supportive for your lower back.

4. Remain here for 5-10 full breath cycles, allowing each exhale to release deeper layers of tension in your lower back and hip.

5. Mindfully release this position before repeating with your left leg, noticing any differences between the two sides.

6. Complete your practice by drawing both knees toward your chest, creating a sense of centeredness and integration.

Corpse Pose (Savasana)

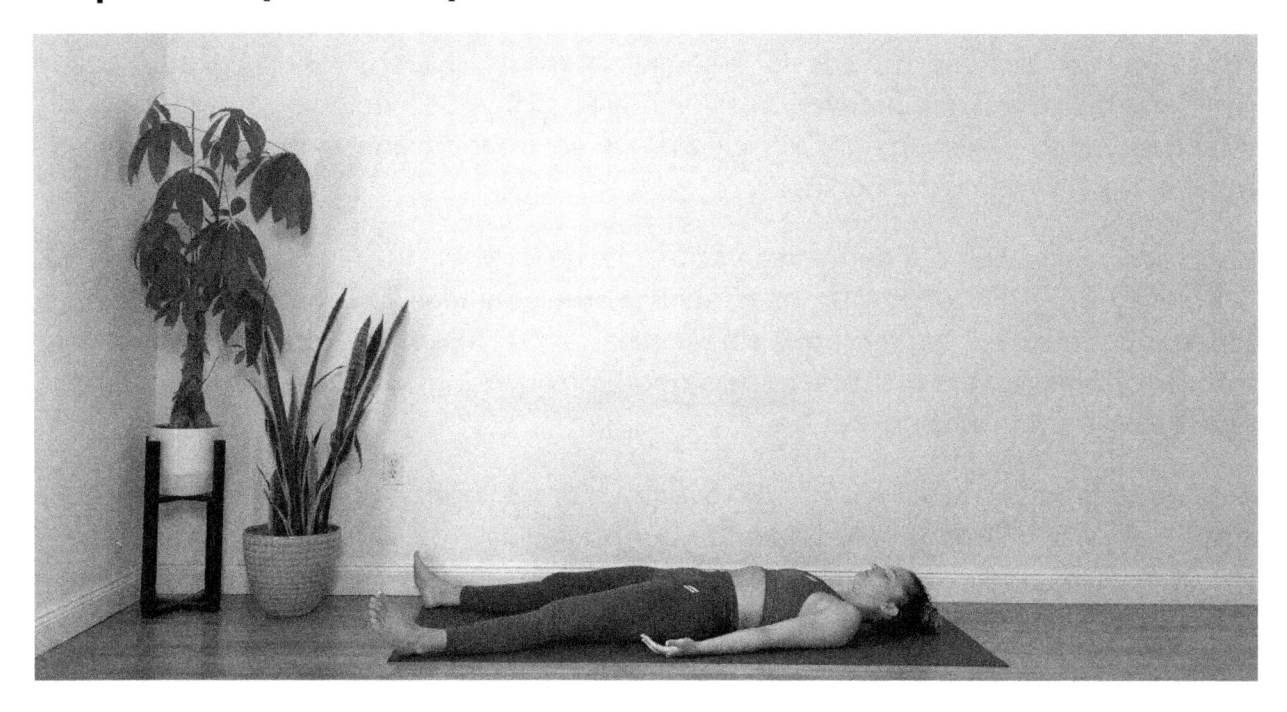

This final resting pose invites complete surrender, allowing your nervous system to integrate the effects of your practice. By deliberately releasing all effort, you're creating space for deep healing and restoration on both physical and energetic levels.

1. Lower yourself to lie on your back, legs extended comfortably with arms resting alongside your body, palms facing upward in a gesture of receptivity.

2. Allow your eyes to close gently, drawing your awareness inward as you take several deep, nourishing breaths.

3. Invite your entire being to release into the support beneath you, surrendering any remaining effort or holding.

4. Either maintain a soft focus on your natural breathing rhythm or conduct a mindful body scan, releasing tension from each area you bring into awareness.

5. Remain in this restorative position for 5-10 minutes, allowing this time of stillness to be as important as the movement that preceded it.

6. When preparing to transition, begin by awakening your fingers and toes with gentle movement, take a deeper breath, and mindfully roll to one side before slowly returning to a seated position.

Foam Rolling for Tension

Foam rolling—aka self-myofascial release—is what happens when a deep-tissue massage and a workout recovery session have a baby. It's a ridiculously simple, wildly effective way to loosen up tight muscles, break up stubborn knots, and keep your body moving like a well-oiled machine.

Your fascia—the web of connective tissue that holds your muscles together—can get stiff, sticky, and downright grumpy, thanks to stress, injuries, or repetitive movements. When that happens, you feel tight, sore, and about as flexible as a two-by-four. Foam rolling applies pressure to these areas, smoothing out adhesions, improving circulation, and giving back your mobility.

And the best part? You're in control. No overpriced massage appointments, no awkward small talk with a stranger digging into your back—just you, a foam roller, and sweet, sweet relief.

Types of Foam Rollers for Tension Release

Not all foam rollers are created equal. Pick the wrong one, and you'll either feel like you're rolling on a pool noodle (useless) or getting steamrolled by a freight train (painful). Here's your cheat sheet:

1. **Smooth, Soft Density Rollers:**

   - Best for: Beginners or anyone who bruises like a peach
   - Feels like: A gentle introduction—like dipping your toe into the foam rolling world
   - Pros: Easy on the muscles, great for full-body rolling
   - Cons: Not aggressive enough if you're dealing with deep knots

2. **Textured or Grid Rollers:**

   - Best for: People who love a good deep tissue massage
   - Feels like: A therapist's knuckles digging into those stubborn trigger points
   - Pros: Gets into tight spots, breaks up knots like a champ
   - Cons: Might be too intense if you're new to this game

3. **Firm Density Rollers:**

   - Best for: Athletes, lifters, and people who don't flinch at the words "deep tissue."

CHAPTER 6: TENSION RELEASE AND TRAUMA MANAGEMENT EXERCISES

- Feels like: A rolling pin flattening out your tight muscles
- Pros: Intense pressure, durable as hell
- Cons: Can be brutal if you're not used to it

4. **Vibrating Foam Rollers:**

   - Best for: Anyone who wants to level up their recovery game
   - Feels like: A foam roller and a muscle relaxer had a high-tech baby
   - Pros: Reduces discomfort, works faster, feels amazing
   - Cons: Pricey, needs charging

5. **Half Rollers or Curved Rollers:**

   - Best for: People with back pain or balance issues
   - Feels like: A more controlled, targeted approach to foam rolling
   - Pros: Great for the spine, won't roll away mid-session
   - Cons: Limited versatility

If you're new to foam rolling, start with a soft-density roller and work your way up. Already used to it? A textured or firm roller will get deeper into those knots. Need the best of the best? A vibrating roller will take your recovery to the next level. Pick the one that suits your pain tolerance, roll out those tight spots, and get back to moving like a human.

Chapter 7: 5-Minute Somatic Exercises

A little progress each day adds up to big results—Satya Nani

For years, the fitness world has been stuck in the "go big or go home" mentality. If you can't dedicate an hour to exercise, why bother at all, right? Wrong. So very wrong.

Think about a regular Tuesday. The to-do list is a mile long, stress levels are through the roof, and the thought of squeezing in an hour-long workout seems as likely as winning the lottery. On days like these, the power of five-minute somatic exercises truly shines. What might seem like nothing at first actually leads to a noticeable shift. Breathing deepens. The knot in your shoulders starts to untangle. At the end of those five minutes, there's a difference. It's not earth-shattering, but it's there—a sense of calm, of being a little more centered.

It's actually doable. Day after day, those five minutes can be found. Sometimes in the morning before the kids wake up, sometimes during a lunch break, and occasionally right before bed. And then, before you even realize it, those little pockets of mindful movement start to add up. Posture improves. Chronic pain eases. Sleep gets better. Turns out consistency trumps intensity every single time. These bite-sized somatic exercises become a secret weapon against stress, a daily reset button. They prove you don't need hours of free time or fancy equipment to make a real difference in how you feel.

So, if you're reading this and thinking, "I don't have time for self-care," the truth is: yes, you do. We all do. In this chapter, we'll explore a variety of five-minute somatic exercises that can seamlessly weave into even the busiest of days. It's all about the small, consistent steps in the right direction. Your body (and mind) will thank you.

5-Minute Somatic Exercise Plans for Anxiety

Grounding Breath and Body Scan

1. **Standing Wall Roll Down (35 sec):** Position back against wall, gradually fold downward vertebra by vertebra, checking for body tightness. Then carefully return upright.

2. **Supine Arm Circles (35 sec):** On your back, create slow circular motions with arms while monitoring shoulder tension. Extra credit for full inhalations.
3. **Lying Hip Release (35 sec):** Recline with knees flexed, allowing them to drop sideways. Direct breath toward any hip or back discomfort.
4. **Somatic Hip Rolls (35 sec):** Remaining reclined, rotate pelvis in deliberate circles, coordinating movement with respiration.
5. **Reclined Butterfly Pose (35 sec):** Connect foot bottoms, let knees spread outward, and direct breath into hip flexor regions.
6. **Seated Side Bend (35 sec):** Sit upright, extend arm sideways, experiencing the lateral stretch through torso. Breathe into expanded areas.
7. **Somatic Scapula Mobilization (35 sec):** In tabletop position, articulate shoulder blades deliberately, matching movements to breath pattern. Supine Knee-to-Chest Pose (35 sec): Draw knees toward torso, experience lumbar relaxation, and breathe completely.

Tension Release Sequence

1. **Cat-Cow Flow (45 sec):** Begin in tabletop position, alternate between lowering chest while curving back (Cow) and lifting spine while dropping head (Cat), timing movements with respiration.
2. **Neck and Shoulder Release (45 sec):** Seated comfortably, drop ear toward shoulder, create slow head rotations, and gently exercise jaw to relieve face tension.
3. **Seated Side Stretch (45 sec):** Sit erect with legs folded, extend one arm upward, bend toward opposite direction, breathe deeply, change sides midway through.
4. **Child's Pose to Cobra Flow (45 sec):** From Child's Pose, glide forward into gentle Cobra, return to starting position, cycle through 3-4 times with breathing.
5. **Bridge Rolls (45 sec):** Recline with knees bent, feet grounded. Gradually lift and lower spine vertebra by vertebra, synchronizing with inhalation and exhalation.
6. **Reclined Twist (45 sec):** While supine, pull knees toward torso, then lower them sideways while gazing opposite, change directions halfway through.
7. **Final Relaxation (30 sec):** Lie supine, progressively release tension from feet to scalp, concentrating on slow, soothing breathing patterns.

Mindful Movement

1. **Standing Star Reach (45 sec):** Begin upright with wide stance, extend arms outward and upward starlike, then bend forward, allowing arms to dangle between feet.
2. **Cat-Cow Pose (45 sec):** In tabletop position, shift between lowering and elevating spine in rhythm with inhalation and exhalation.
3. **Thread the Needle (45 sec):** Starting on all fours, slide one arm underneath opposite arm, resting lateral shoulder and face on floor, switch sides.
4. **Child's Pose with Side Stretch (45 sec):** Kneel with buttocks on heels, extend arms rightward then leftward for gentle lateral extensions.
5. **Gentle Bridge Lifts (45 sec):** Recline supine, knees flexed, feet planted. Smoothly elevate and lower pelvis coordinating with breath.
6. **Final Twist (45 sec):** Rest on back, direct bent knees to one side, arms extended perpendicular to body, rotate to opposite side midway.

Calming Hand and Foot Focus

1. **Hand Massage (2 min):** Slowly knead both hands, concentrating on tactile feedback.
2. **Foot Rolls (1 min):** Rotate each foot across a small sphere or against the ground.
3. **Finger Tapping (2 min):** Methodically touch each digit to thumb, attending to cadence and feeling.

5-Minute Somatic Exercise Plans for Stress

Breath and Spine Release

1. **Somatic Wave (35 sec):** In tabletop position, flow spine in rippling motions from sacrum to crown, matching movement with slow, rhythmic respiration.
2. **Standing Wall Roll Down (35 sec):** With back to wall, fold down and rise vertebra by vertebra, directing breath into each spinal section during movement.
3. **Somatic Sunbird Pose (35 sec):** From all fours, raise opposing limbs outward, inhale into spinal elongation, alternate sides with each breath cycle.
4. **Dynamic Bridge Pose (35 sec):** Supine, elevate and lower spine with respiration, ascending during inhalation, descending with exhalation, moving deliberately.

5. **Seated Side Bend (35 sec):** Sitting cross-legged, stretch arm upward and lean laterally, creating vertebral spacing through breath, switch directions.
6. **Somatic Cobra Pose (35 sec):** From belly, subtly raise sternum while inhaling, lower while exhaling, emphasizing individual vertebral movement.
7. **Reclined Spinal Twist (35 sec):** Lying supine, knees directed sideways, arms extended, breathe into spinal rotation, change sides midway through.
8. **Knees to Chest Rocking (35 sec):** Embrace knees toward torso, sway gently sideways, massaging back while sustaining deep, consistent breathing patterns.

Grounding and Releasing

1. **Foot Press (1 min):** Rise and push different foot surfaces against floor, noticing the contact points.
2. **Palm Presses (1 min):** Join hands at heart center, adjusting force. Concentrate on tactile awareness.
3. **Standing Forward Bend (2 min):** Fold forward from hip joints, releasing upper limbs and head downward. Rock subtly.
4. **Gentle Backbend (1 min):** Upright with palms supporting lumbar region. Slightly curve spine backward, attending to respiration

Tension Melting Sequence

1. **Somatic Tabletop Cat-Cow (45 sec):** In quadruped position, shift between lowering and lifting spine with inhalation and exhalation, moving deliberately and consciously.
2. **Butterfly Release (45 sec):** Seated with foot bottoms touching, knees apart. Rhythmically press knees downward maintaining elongated spine, then tilt forward slightly.
3. **Hip Circles (45 sec):** Remaining seated, legs extended wide, palms planted behind, create gradual circular motions with upper body to ease lumbar region.
4. **Knee to Chest Rocking (45 sec):** Supine, draw knees toward sternum and sway gently side-to-side, providing spinal massage.
5. **Reclined Figure-4 (45 sec):** While supine, place right ankle across left leg, clasp hands behind left thigh. Alternate midway through.
6. **Reclined Spinal Twist (45 sec):** On back, pull knees toward chest, then lower them sideways while rotating head oppositely. Alternate sides.

7. **Corpse Pose with Progressive Release (30 sec):** Lie flat, methodically relaxing tensions from feet to crown with each exhalation.

Mindful Stretching

1. **Seated Side Stretch (2 min):** Sit with crossed legs. Extend one arm upward, then bend toward opposite direction. Switch sides.
2. **Seated Twist (2 min):** Seated with straight legs. Flex one knee and position opposing elbow outside the bent knee. Rotate gently. Alternate sides.
3. **Child's Pose (1 min):** From kneeling, rest buttocks on heels, reach arms forward. Notice the extension along your spine.

Energy Shift

1. **Half Moon Pose (40 sec):** Balance on one leg, extend the other horizontally while reaching one arm to the floor and the other skyward, creating a stellar alignment.
2. **Warrior II Pulses (35 sec):** Stand with legs wide, front knee bent, arms extended. Pulse deeper into the pose with each breath, maintaining strong alignment.
3. **Standing Tree Flow (35 sec):** Balance on one foot, place opposite foot against standing leg, flow arms overhead like branches, switch sides halfway through.
4. **Extended Side Angle (35 sec):** From warrior stance, lower one arm to floor beside front foot, extend other arm overhead creating a long diagonal line.
5. **Eagle Arms with Forward Fold (35 sec):** Cross arms at elbows, fold forward from hips, allowing wrapped arms to hang heavily, breathing into upper back.
6. **Standing Pigeon (35 sec):** Balance on one leg, cross other ankle above knee, sit back as if lowering into a chair, fold forward slightly.
7. **Triangle Pose Flows (35 sec):** Legs wide, extend torso sideways, lower hand toward ankle, reach opposite arm upward, flow between sides with breath.
8. **Standing Forward Bend with Shoulder Opener (30 sec):** Fold forward from hips, interlace hands behind back, allow arms to float overhead, releasing shoulder tension.

5-Minute Somatic Exercise Plans for Trauma

Grounding and Present-Moment Awareness Sequence

1. **Standing Wall Roll Down (35 sec):** Position yourself upright against wall. Gradually fold downward vertebra by vertebra, allowing arms and head to

dangle. Then, carefully return to standing.

2. **Somatic Hip Rolls (35 sec):** Recline with knees bent, feet grounded. Create deliberate circular motions with pelvis, letting spine respond naturally. Reverse direction midway.

3. **Somatic Wave (35 sec):** In tabletop position, create undulating movement beginning at tailbone flowing through spine, coordinating motion with respiration.

4. **Dynamic Warrior I (35 sec):** Position one foot backward into lunge, arms extended upward. Rhythmically lower rear knee while reaching higher. Alternate sides.

5. **Somatic Side Stretch (35 sec):** Stand feet aligned with hips. Lift one arm overhead, gently elongating lateral torso with subtle pulsing movements. Alternate sides.

6. **Seated Side Bend (35 sec):** Sit legs crossed, extend one arm upward, bend toward opposite direction. Pulse softly while breathing into ribcage. Alternate sides.

7. **Somatic Scapula Mobilization (35 sec):** From all fours, draw shoulder blades together, then separate them apart using slow, deliberate control.

8. **Supine Knee-to-Chest Pose (35 sec):** Lying supine, draw knees toward chest, create small circular movements massaging lower spine. Change direction halfway through.

Breath and Movement Connection Sequence

1. **Supine Arm Circles (35 sec):** Recline on back and create circular arm motions, breathing in as they ascend, breathing out as they descend. Experiment with different diameters.

2. **Dynamic Bridge Pose (35 sec):** While supine, knees flexed, inhale as you elevate pelvis, exhale during descent, moving rhythmically with respiration.

3. **Somatic Wave (35 sec):** In tabletop position, generate subtle spinal undulation, inhaling during forward movement, exhaling when shifting backward.

4. **Chair Pose with Arm Waves (35 sec):** Lower into seated hover and perform flowing, undulating arm movements, coordinating with breath cycles.

5. **Standing Spinal Wave (35 sec):** Flex knees slightly and create wavelike spinal movement from cranium to coccyx, allowing breath to guide motion.

6. **Somatic Chest Opener (35 sec):** Whether seated or upright, broaden chest during inhalation, subtly retracting scapulae. Release with exhalation.

CHAPTER 7: 5-MINUTE SOMATIC EXERCISES

7. **Child's Pose with Arm Walks (35 sec):** In folded position, extend arms forward while inhaling, retract while exhaling, establishing consistent breathing rhythm.

8. **Somatic Shoulder Bridge (35 sec):** Lying supine, knees bent, raise and lower hips synchronizing with breath, articulating each spinal segment during transition.

Safe Space Visualization and Anchoring

1. **Supine Arm Circles (35 sec):** Recline on back, creating gradual circular motions with arms while envisioning a sheltering radiance encompassing your body.

2. **Child's Pose with Arm Walks (35 sec):** Fold into child's pose, extending arms forward, imagining anchoring tendrils connecting downward with each stretch.

3. **Reclined Butterfly Pose (35 sec):** Allow knees to relax outward, visualizing a protective envelope of warmth and security surrounding you.

4. **Somatic Hip Rolls (35 sec):** Lying supine, knees flexed, rotate pelvis in deliberate circles, imagining yourself nestled in gentle support.

5. **Seated Side Bend (35 sec):** Extend one arm skyward and tilt laterally as though creating a defensive curve around your form.

6. **Somatic Scapula Mobilization (35 sec):** In tabletop position, articulate shoulder blades as if expanding and contracting protective feathered appendages.

7. **Lying Hip Release (35 sec):** Allow knees to drift side to side while picturing yourself within a tranquil haven.

8. **Corpse Pose (35 sec):** Stretch out completely, sensing complete earth support, embraced by a sphere of security and profound restoration.

Important Notes:

- Move at your own pace—there's no rush.
- If anything feels uncomfortable, pause or modify.
- Breathe slowly and steadily—your breath is your anchor.
- If emotions arise, let them come and go without judgment.
- These exercises help you reconnect with your body in a safe, gentle way.
- If you're working with a therapist, consider discussing these practices with them.

EPILOGUE

I'm learning to be with what's alive in me, moment by moment. To prioritize rest in a world that glorifies burnout. To slow down the pace of my nervous system instead of racing to keep up with a society that treats exhaustion like a badge of honor.

Imagine a Monday morning in a crowded coffee shop and caffeine-fueled mayhem fills the air, with cups clattering, espresso machines yelling, and people acting as though they like early meetings. A woman sits quietly with her eyes closed amid everything. Is she sleeping? Nope. She's tuned in. Hands resting on her lap, breath deep and steady. She's not zoning out—she's dropping in.

Variations of this moment happen everywhere, every day. The office worker pausing to unclench his jaw before a meeting. The teenager flopping onto their bed, feeling their breath settle after an overstimulating day. The old man stretching in the park, moving like someone who understands that his body is worth listening to.

These aren't dramatic, headline-worthy acts. No one's throwing a parade because you finally unclenched your shoulders. But these moments? They're everything. Because each one is a tiny rebellion against the noise, a refusal to ignore the body's quiet intelligence.

For some, this journey is a slow burn—like turning up the volume on a song that's been playing in the background for years. For others, it's a sudden realization: "Oh, THIS is what it means to be in my body." And sure, old habits don't disappear overnight. Society isn't going to stop rewarding busyness just because you decided to breathe more deeply. But with each pause, each check-in, each moment of radical self-awareness, a new pattern takes shape.

This book is not a finish line.

It's a call to continue investing To continue listening. And, to keep coming back to oneself. Because there is always a way to return home—to your body, your breath, and your wisdom—no matter how hectic life becomes. The next time deadlines overwhelm you, you're doom scrolling, or you're just trying to survive in this crazy world, take a pause. Close your eyes. Breathe. Listen carefully. Because your body has been telling a story all along—a story of vitality, intelligence, and tenacity.

That story is still unfolding, one mindful moment at a time.

Here's to moving at the speed of our nervous systems, resting when we need to, and celebrating the absolute genius of our bodies. Because they know the way home. We just have to listen.

EXERCISE LIST

Arch and Flatten	39
Body Scan	40
Body Scan Meditation	75
Cat-Cow Pose (Marjaryasana-Bitilasana)	32
Chair Pose with Arm Waves	68
Child's Pose with Arm Walks	90
Constructive Rest Position	38
Corpse Pose (Savasana)	99
Dynamic Bridge Pose	94
Dynamic Child's Pose (Balasana) with Arm Reaches	33
Dynamic Downward Dog	70
Dynamic Tree Pose	66
Dynamic Warrior I	63
Gentle Neck Rolls	37
Gentle Standing Twists	65
Grounding Techniques	41
Knees to Chest Rocking	97
Loving-Kindness Meditation (Metta)	74
Lying Hip Release	60
Meditation and Mindfulness Practices	73
Mindfulness Meditation	74
Pelvic Tilts	36
Physical Grounding:	41
Progressive Muscle Relaxation	40
Reclined Butterfly Pose	72
Reclined Hamstring Stretch	86
Reclined Spinal Twist	93
Seated Arm Circles	84
Seated Figure Four Stretch	83
Seated Forward Fold with Rocking	80
Seated Side Bend	82
Side-Lying Leg Lifts	45
Somatic Chest Opener	84
Somatic Cobra Pose	88
Somatic Crescent Lunge	71
Somatic Forward Fold	67
Somatic Frog Pose	86

Somatic Half-Bow Pose	89
Somatic Hip Rolls	59
Somatic Pigeon Pose	92
Somatic Scapula Mobilization	91
Somatic Shoulder Bridge	96
Somatic Shoulder Shrugs	46
Somatic Side Stretch	69
Somatic Sunbird Pose	58
Somatic Twists	42
Somatic Warrior II	64
Somatic Wave	61
Sphinx Pose	44
Spinal Rolls (Seated or Standing)	34
Standing Pelvic Tilts	62
Standing Spinal Wave	95
Standing Wall Roll Down	56
Steps for Standing Spinal Rolls:	35
Supine Arm Circles	57
Supine Knee-to-Chest Pose (Apanasana)	98
Tabletop Arm and Leg Extensions	43
Thread The Needle	81

ADDITIONAL READING

10 somatic interventions explained—integrative psychotherapy mental health blog. (n.d.). Integrative Psychotherapy & Trauma Treatment. https://integrativepsych.co/new-blog/somatic-therapy-explained-methods

Aybar, S. (2021, July 21). *4 at-home somatic therapy exercises for trauma recovery.* Psych Central. https://psychcentral.com/lib/somatic-therapy-exercises-for-trauma

Babauta, L. (n.d.). *How to make exercise a daily habit: Zen habits.* Zenhabits.net. https://zenhabits.net/how-to-make-exercise-a-daily-habit-with-a-may-challenge/

Babuta, L. (2017, February 10). *Letting go of distractions.* Zen Habits. https://zenhabits.net/distractions/

Blanton, K. (2024, February 28). *Somatic stretching may be the gentle workout you've been waiting for—What to know.* Prevention. https://www.prevention.com/fitness/workouts/a46993501/somatic-exercises/

Burnett-Zeigler, I., Schuette, S., Victorson, D., & Wisner, K. L. (2016). Mind–Body approaches to treating mental health symptoms among disadvantaged populations: A comprehensive review. *Journal of Alternative and Complementary Medicine, 22*(2), 115–124. https://doi.org/10.1089/acm.2015.0038

Burton, N. (2022, November 16). *7 somatic stretching exercises for flexibility and stress relief.* DailyOM.com. https://www.dailyom.com/journal/7-somatic-stretching-exercises-for-flexibility-and-stress-relief/

Byrne, C. (2022, September 22). *Somatic stretching: How it works, benefits, and getting started.* Everyday Health. https://www.everydayhealth.com/fitness/what-is-somatic-stretching/

Chair cat-cow pose yoga (chair Marjaryasana Bitilasana). (2017, October 15). Tummee.com. https://www.tummee.com/yoga-poses/chair-cat-cow-pose

Conlon, K. (2021, March 25). *5 Trauma release exercises you can try at home!* Cohesive Therapy NYC. https://cohesivetherapynyc.com/blog/5-trauma-release-exercises-you-can-try-at-home/

Cronkleton, E. (2019, April 9). *10 breathing techniques.* Healthline. https://www.healthline.com/health/breathing-exercise

Cuncic, A. (2019). *Chill out: How to use progressive muscle relaxation to quell anxiety.* Verywell Mind. https://www.verywellmind.com/how-do-i-practice-progressive-muscle-relaxation-3024400

Dropping anchor: an ACT skill. (2021, September 24). Flourish Mindfully. https://www.flourishmindfully.com.au/blog/dropping-anchor

Dubois-Maahs, J. (2020, October 16). *What is somatic therapy, and how can it benefit you?* Talkspace. https://www.talkspace.com/blog/somatic-therapy-what-is-definition-get-started-guide/

Dunbar, T. (2021, December 8). *The 5 keys to unlocking consistency.* Curious. https://medium.com/curious/the-5-keys-to-unlocking-consistency-c9f730c47b3b

Eleanor, M. (2022, April 25). *10 types of energy healing: Which one is right for you?* LocallyWell. https://www.locallywell.com/10-types-of-energy-healing-which-one-is-right-for-you/

Extended triangle pose (utthita trikonasana). (2007, August 28). Yoga Journal. https://www.yogajournal.com/poses/extended-triangle-pose/

Fargo, S. (2020, August 26). *Mindfulness body scan for gratitude.* Mindfulness Exercises. https://mindfulnessexercises.com/mindfulness-body-scan-for-gratitude/

Fitzpatrick, T. (2020, October 10). *Relax & release lower back pain sequence.* Alignsomatics.com. https://www.alignsomatics.com/blog/relax-release-lower-back-pain-sequence

Foster, L. (2023, May 16). *How to choose the right gym for you: A comprehensive guide.* Educate Fitness. https://educatefitness.co.uk/how-to-choose-the-right-gym-for-you-a-comprehensive-guide/

Gallo, A. (2023, February 15). *What is psychological safety?* Harvard Business Review. https://hbr.org/2023/02/what-is-psychological-safety

Half-moon pose with chair yoga (Ardha Chandrasana with chair) | yoga sequences, benefits, variations, and Sanskrit pronunciation. (2019, September 17). Tummee. https://www.tummee.com/yoga-poses/half-moon-pose-with-chair

Headache exercise. (n.d.). Somatic Movement Center. Retrieved March 27, 2024, from https://somaticmovementcenter.com/headache-exercise/

Huang, Q., & AmaniAli Babgi. (2022). Effect of Hanna somatic education on low back and neck pain levels. *Saudi Journal of Medicine and Medical Sciences, 10*(3), 266–266. https://doi.org/10.4103/sjmms.sjmms_580_21

Improving your body image. (2020, May 21). National Alliance for Eating Disorders. https://www.allianceforeatingdisorders.com/5-secrets-positive-body-image/

Kristen Van Bael, Ball, M., Scarfo, J., & Emra Suleyman. (2023). Assessment of the mind-body connection: preliminary psychometric evidence for a new self-report questionnaire. *BMC Psychology, 11*(1). https://doi.org/10.1186/s40359-023-01302-3

Lockart, E. (2023, March 27). *What is grounding, and can it help improve your health?* Healthline. https://www.healthline.com/health/grounding

Lynning, M., Svane, C., Westergaard, K., Bergien, S. O., Gunnersen, S. R., & Skovgaard, L. (2021). Tension and trauma releasing exercises for people with multiple sclerosis – An exploratory pilot study. *Journal of Traditional and Complementary Medicine, 11*(5), 383–389. https://doi.org/10.1016/j.jtcme.2021.02.003

Mcphillips, K. (2020, February 20). *"Somatic exercises" stretch the stress right out of your poor, aching body.* Well+Good. https://www.wellandgood.com/somatic-exercises/

Mehling, W. E., Wrubel, J., Daubenmier, J. J., Price, C. J., Kerr, C. E., Silow, T., Gopisetty, V., & Stewart, A. L. (2011). Body Awareness: a phenomenological inquiry into the common ground of mind-body therapies. *Philosophy, Ethics, and Humanities in Medicine, 6*(1), 6. https://doi.org/10.1186/1747-5341-6-6

Miller, A. (2018). *10 Ways to use sensory experiences to build mindfulness.* Happify. https://www.happify.com/hd/use-sensory-experiences-to-build-mindfulness/

Nesci, N. (2020, March 4). *5 things everyone needs to know about energy healing.* The Growth & Wellness Therapy Centre. https://www.growthwellnesstherapy.com/our-blog/5-things-everyone-needs-to-know-about-energy-healing

Oschman, J., Chevalier, G., & Brown, R. (2015). The effects of grounding (earthing) on inflammation, the immune response, wound healing, and prevention and treatment of chronic inflammatory and autoimmune diseases. *Journal of Inflammation Research, 8*, 83. https://doi.org/10.2147/jir.s69656

Ragdoll. (2019, May 11). Yoga 15. https://yoga15.com/pose/ragdoll/

Recovery from trauma and the mind-body connection. (2023, May 9). Newport Institute. https://www.newportinstitute.com/resources/mental-health/the-mind-body-connection/

Scott, E. (2023, August 23). *How to create a "safe space" anyplace.* Verywell Mind. https://www.verywellmind.com/how-and-why-you-should-create-a-safe-space-for-yourself-3144981

Shaking meditation: The easiest way to release stress in five minutes. (2019, November 19). *The Times of India.* https://timesofindia.indiatimes.com/life-style/health-fitness/home-remedies/shaking-meditation-the-easiest-way-to-release-stress-in-five-minutes/articleshow/72127094.cms

Stelter, G. (2018, September 20). *Trap stretches: Loosen your trapezius muscles*. Healthline. https://www.healthline.com/health/fitness-exercise/trapezius-stretches

Surles, T. (2023, March 15). *Exercising for better sleep: 5 reasons it works*. Healthline. https://www.healthline.com/health/5-reasons-exercise-improves-sleep

Toussaint, L., Nguyen, Q. A., Roettger, C., Dixon, K., Offenbächer, M., Kohls, N., Hirsch, J., & Sirois, F. (2021). Effectiveness of progressive muscle relaxation, deep breathing, and guided imagery in promoting psychological and physiological states of relaxation. *Evidence-Based Complementary and Alternative Medicine, 2021*(1), 1–8. https://doi.org/10.1155/2021/5924040

Tummee.com. (2024a). *Seated tree pose foot side chair yoga (Upavistha Vrksasana pada parsva chair) | yoga sequences, benefits, variations, and sanskrit pronunciation*. Tummee.com. https://www.tummee.com/yoga-poses/seated-tree-pose-foot-side-chair

Tummee.com. (2024b). *Seated warrior pose I chair (upavistha virabhadrasana I chair) variations - 47 variations of seated warrior pose I chair | tummee.com*. Tummee. https://www.tummee.com/yoga-poses/seated-warrior-pose-i-chair/variations

Upadhayay, P. (2023, February 1). *How to incorporate yoga into your daily routine*. Hindustan Times. https://www.hindustantimes.com/lifestyle/health/how-to-incorporate-yoga-into-your-daily-routine-101674626859419.html

Warrior II pose (Virabhadrasana II). (2007, August 28). Yoga Journal. https://www.yogajournal.com/poses/warrior-ii-pose/

What is Utthita chaturanga dandasana? (n.d.). Yogapedia. Retrieved March 10, 2024, from https://www.yogapedia.com/definition/10670/utthita-chaturanga-dandasana

Printed in Dunstable, United Kingdom